I0440868

Developing Prize Winning Abdominals

by Doug Brolus

ISBN-10: 148392405X
ISBN-13: 978-1483924052

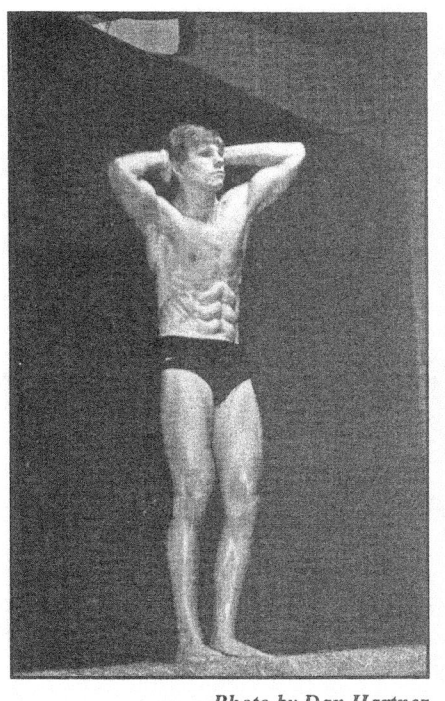

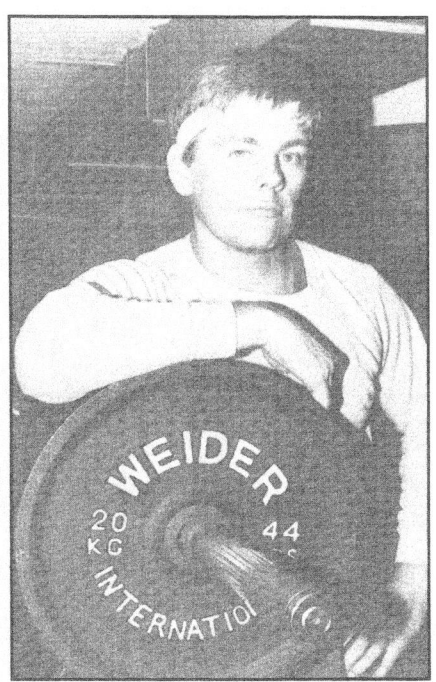

Photo by Dan Hartner　　　　　　　　　　　　*Photo by Tom Mobley*

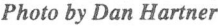

DOUG BROLUS

Height: 6′ 1½″

Weight: 190

Chest: 46

Waist: 32

Arms: 16

Neck: 16

Thigh: 24

Calves: 16

Body Building Titles Won

Teenage Mr. Michigan - Best Abdominals
Teenage Mr. Wolverine - 3rd Place

Contests I have competed in:

Teenage Mr. Michigan Highlands
Jr. Mr. Michigan
Mr. Great Lakes
Michigan Natural Body Building Championships

Movie Credit

I played a boxer in the movie "Tough Enough" -
20th Century Fox Film

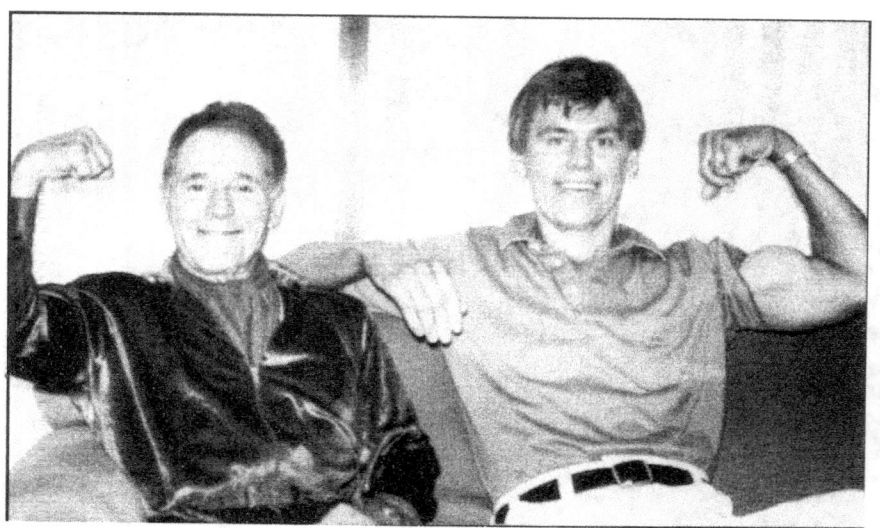

Here I am pictured with my friend Jack LaLanne, one of the greatest bodybuilders of all time, who helped me in my training and diet. Jack LaLanne was the inventor the leg extension machine, the weight selector pin machines and the first cable machine. Jack was the father of the fitness movement in the USA and Jack is known around the world for his feats of strength and his TV exercise show.

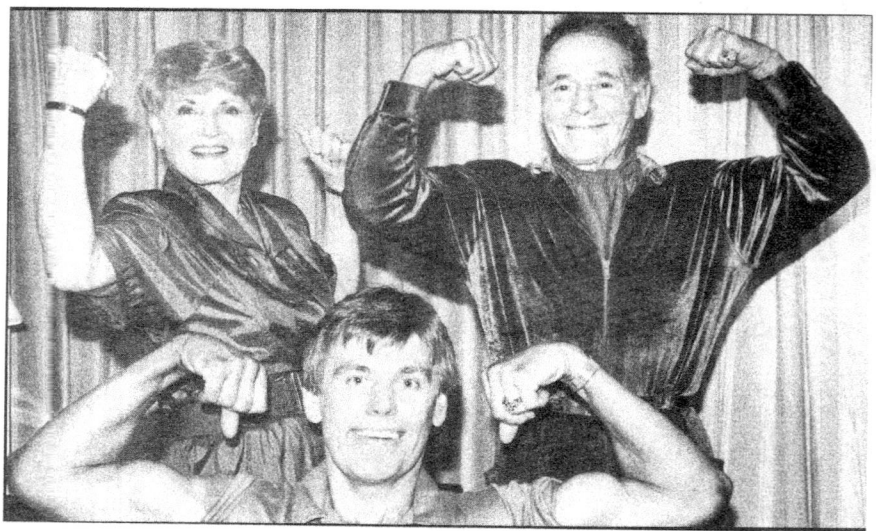

I am pictured with Jack LaLanne and his wife Elaine.

Photos by Leon Bach

Special thanks

I would like to extend a thank you to everyone who has helped and supported me throughout all my years in bodybuilding.

Ironman Magazine

Thanks to Steve Holman, Editor of Ironman Magazine for all his help. Steve is one of the best writers in bodybuilding and has a great knowledge of fitness and diet.

Thanks to the publisher of Ironman, John Balik, one of the greatest publishers and photographers.

I would like to thank Leon Bach, one of the greatest physique photographers, for taking many of the fantastic photos in my booklet. Leon worked for Ironman Magazine.

Thanks to Joe Weider, founder and former publisher of Muscle and Fitness, for his help.

A special note of appreciation for Jack LaLanne for his help with my training and diet, for his friendship and inspiration. Jack has since passed on but his fitness legacy lives.

Thanks to Eddie Giuliani for all his help and thanks to Zabo.

Thanks to Dave Draper, Movie Star, Mr. Universe and Mr. World for all his help.

Thanks to Steve Douglas, photographer, for Musclemag International, and the staff for all their help.

Thanks to Ron Kosloff, owner of NSP.

Thanks to William and Norman Dabish who own Powerhouse Gym.

Contributing Photographers
Leon Bach - Ironman Magazine
Dave Siegle - Hollywood, California - Cover Shot
Tom Mobley
Dan Hartner
Paula Crane

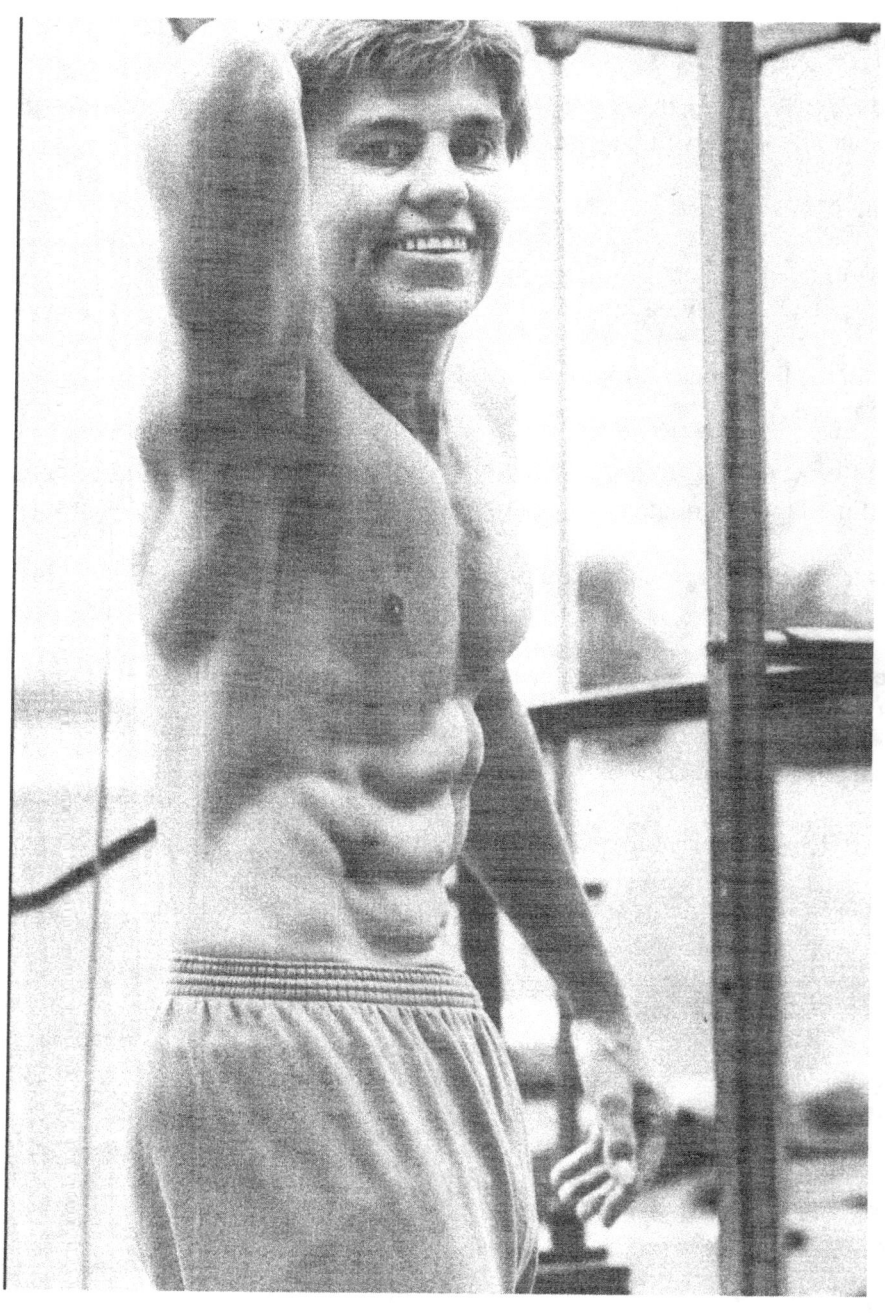

You have to watch your diet all year long if you want a great set of abs. This shot shows the Serratus, Intercostals, External Obliques and Rectus Abdominals.

Photo by Leon Bach at World Gym in Venice, California

Tips on training and diet

The stomach muscles are one of the most impressive groups of muscles when properly developed. The muscles that make up the entire waist are the Rectus Abdominals, which cover the front part of the waist. The muscles that are at the side of the waist are the External Oblique, the Serratus and Intercostals. Each of the these muscles must be exercised separately if you expect to develop them equally.

You must not develop one area of the waist more than another. Balance is the key in training the waist or any other muscle group. Train the abdominal muscles four days a week. I suggest training the waist Tuesday, Wednesday, Friday and Saturday. Exercising the waist will keep the muscles firm, and following a good diet at the same time will help you get the results you want. Getting clear cut definition is eighty percent diet and twenty percent exercise. The benefits of having a good waistline are improved digestion and better posture because the abdominals help keep the back straight. Your overall health will improve because all the training helps keep the internal organs in great functional condition with all the blood being pumped into the region.

Serratus, Intercostals, Obliques

The abdominal muscles command attention when they are highly developed and have very little adipose tissue on them. To have the look of a true champion, the Serratus, Intercostals and Obliques should be developed to the point where it looks like little fingers on the sides of the waist. The key in abdominal training is balance. The abs, including the rectus abdominus, should be thick and deeply cut. This is the look for which to strive. It takes a lot of hard training and adherence to a good diet low in fat all year long. Stay away from bulk up diets and trying to cut back a few weeks before a contest or you will end up with less muscle size and too much fat on the abs. If you watch your diet all year long you can peak out for a contest very fast with no trouble.

Diet is about 80% and training is about 20% of the abdominal appearance. If you want cut abs, cut back on the fat in the diet. Keep the reps high on the abdominal exercises and use little weight for each exercise. Do not rest too long between sets; keep a good pace. The abs respond very well when trained four days a week. Change the exercises around - this will help keep your motivation up. The stronger the abdominals are, the better you will feel. The abs keep your body in an upright positions and also help your digestion work to its optimum ability. Flexing the abs after every training session will help get better control and flexibility.

Train hard and follow a food diet - the rest will come fast. Do sit ups and leg lifts on a bench for the rectus abdominals.

This is the program; now get started and look for the great results!

EXERCISES

Serratus, Intercostals, Obliques

Cable Pulls

The first exercise you should start with is cable pulls. Bend down on the floor with the knees, grab a V grip pulley handle and pull the weight down toward you and touch the floor. When the hand touches the floor, squeeze the serratus muscles. Exercise will make the serratus stand out like fingers on the lateral part of the waist. Try doing 3 sets of 20 reps on this exercise.

Trunk Twists

The second exercise will be seated trunk twists with an empty weight lifting bar. Sit on a roman chair or a bench press, put the bar behind the neck and let it rest on the traps. Twist back and forth at a fast pace.

This exercise will help develop the intercostals and the external obliques: Try doing 1 set of 100 to 200 reps. This exercise is very easy to perform and very effective.

Side Bends

The third exercise is side bends with a light dumbbell. Take a dumbbell in one hand and put your other hand on the back of your head and rock back and forth. Squeeze the intercostals and obliques each time you move your torso. Switch hands and do the other side. This exercise will help give the muscles deep and thick cuts. One set of 50 to 100 reps each side.

Anatomy and Physiology of the Serratus, Intercostals, Obliques

Muscle: Serratus
Origin: Ribs (upper eight or nine)
Insertion: Scapula anterior surface, vertebral border
Function: Pulls shoulder forward, abducts and rotates it upward
Innervation: Long Thoracic nerve

Muscle: Intercostals
Origin: Rib lower border forward fibers
Insertion: Rib upper border of rib below origin
Function: Elevate ribs
Innervation: Lower seven intercostal nerves and iliohypogastric nerves

Muscle: Oblique
Origin: Rib (lower eight)
Insertion: Ossa coxal iliac crest and pubis by way of inguinal ligament
Function: Compress abdomen, important postural function of all abdominal muscles is to pull front of pelvis upward thereby flattening lumbar curve of spine. When these muscles lose their tone, common figure faults of protruding abdomen and lordosis develop.

Knowing where a muscle is and how it functions will help you in your training.

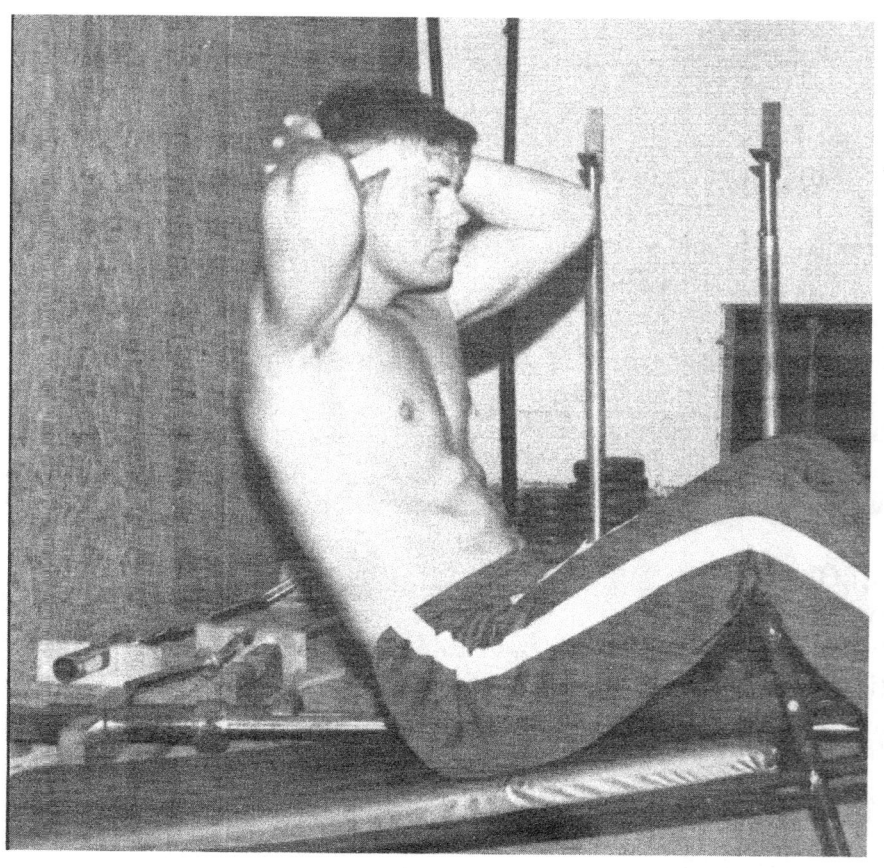

SIT UPS

This is a great exercise to develop the upper abdominals. Lay down on a sit up board, bend your knees and bring your upper body all the way up. Do 3 sets of 10 reps to start with. Do as many reps each set as you want when you are able to. Put a 10 pound weight plate behind your head wrapped in a towel or cushion for extra resistance.

Photo by Tom Mobley

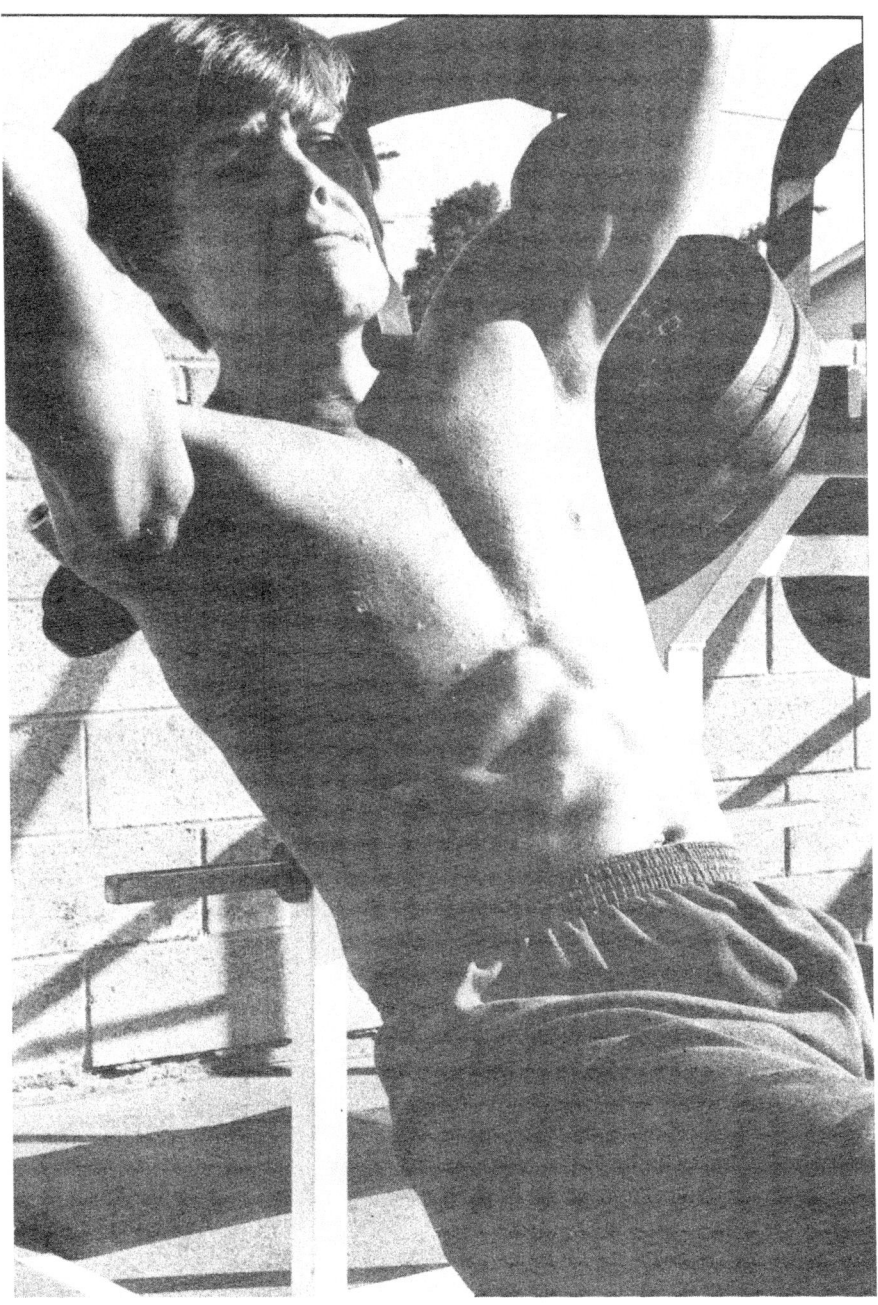

Roman Chair Sit-ups are one of the best exercises for the front abdominals. Go back ½ way on the bench and come all the way back up. If you don't have a Roman Chair, sit up on a bench and have somebody hold your feet. To be most effective, this exercise should be done with high repetitions.

Photo by Leon Bach at World Gym in Venice, California

by DOUG BROLUS

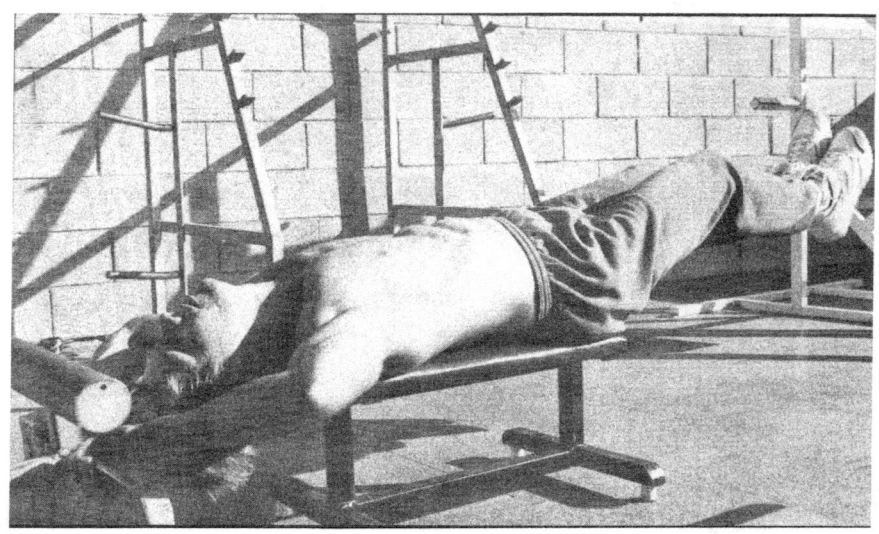

Leg Lifts On Bench

Lay down on a bench. Lift your legs ¾ way up and let the legs down even with the bench. Do not let the feet touch the floor. This exercise will strengthen the lower abdominals.

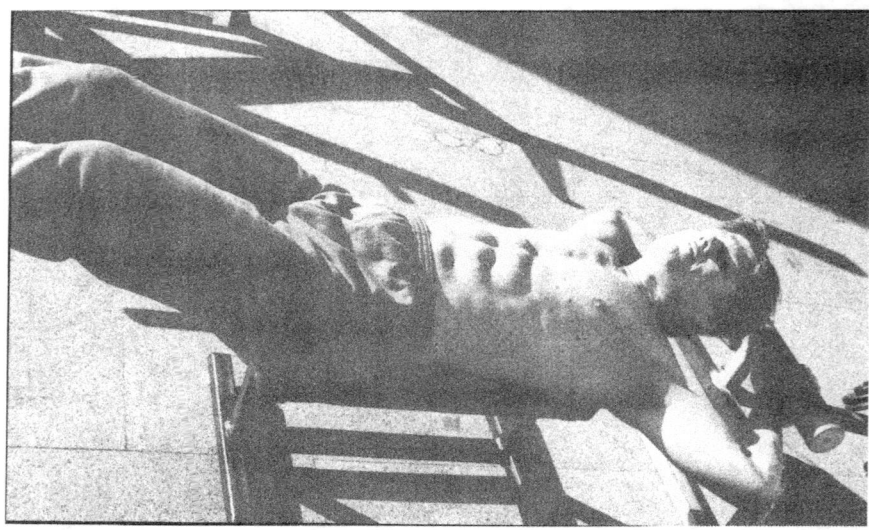

This exercise is great for the upper and lower abdominals. Do a high number of reps on each set.

Photo by Leon Bach at World Gym in Venice, California

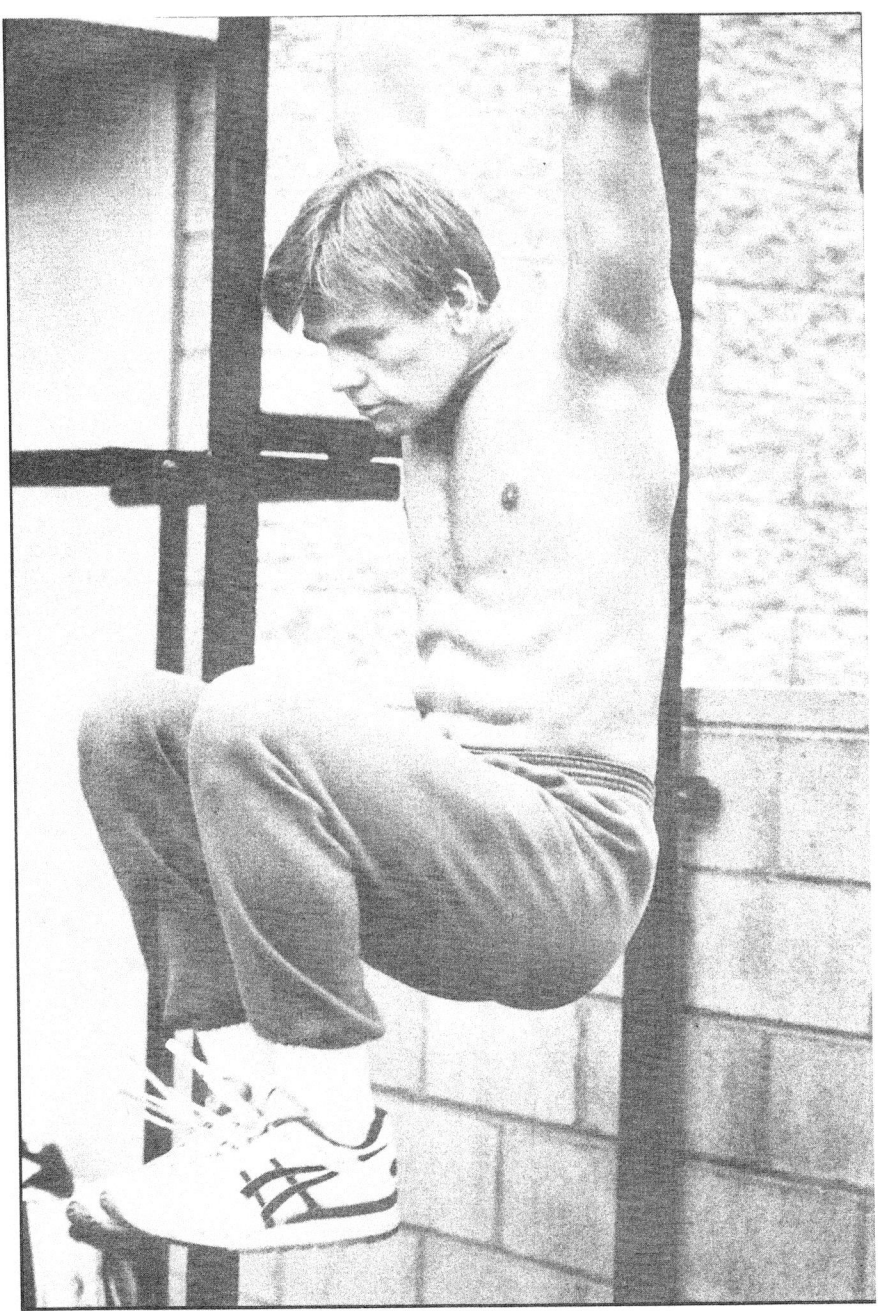

Hanging Leg Raises Bent Knee: Grip a chinning bar and bring your knees to your chest and let your knees back down. This exercise will strengthen the whole abdominal area. Do as many repetitions of each set as you feel you can.

Photo by Leon Bach at World Gym in Venice, California

by DOUG BROLUS

11

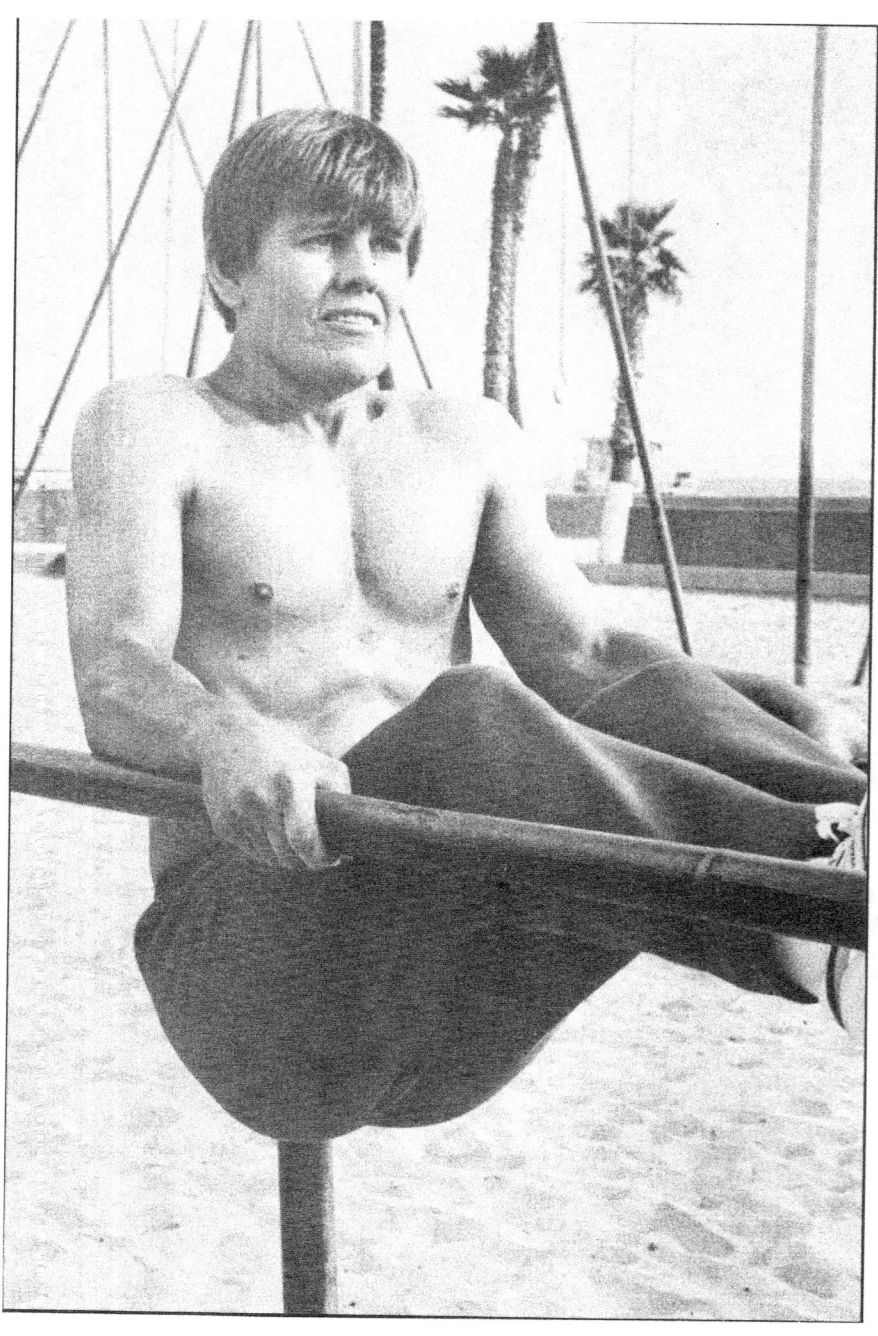

Leg lifts on the dip bars are beneficial for the upper & lower abdominals and also have a great effect on the Serratus & Intercostals. Do 3 sets of as many reps as you want.

Photo by Leon Bach at World Gym in Venice, California

DEVELOPING PRIZE WINNING ABDOMINALS

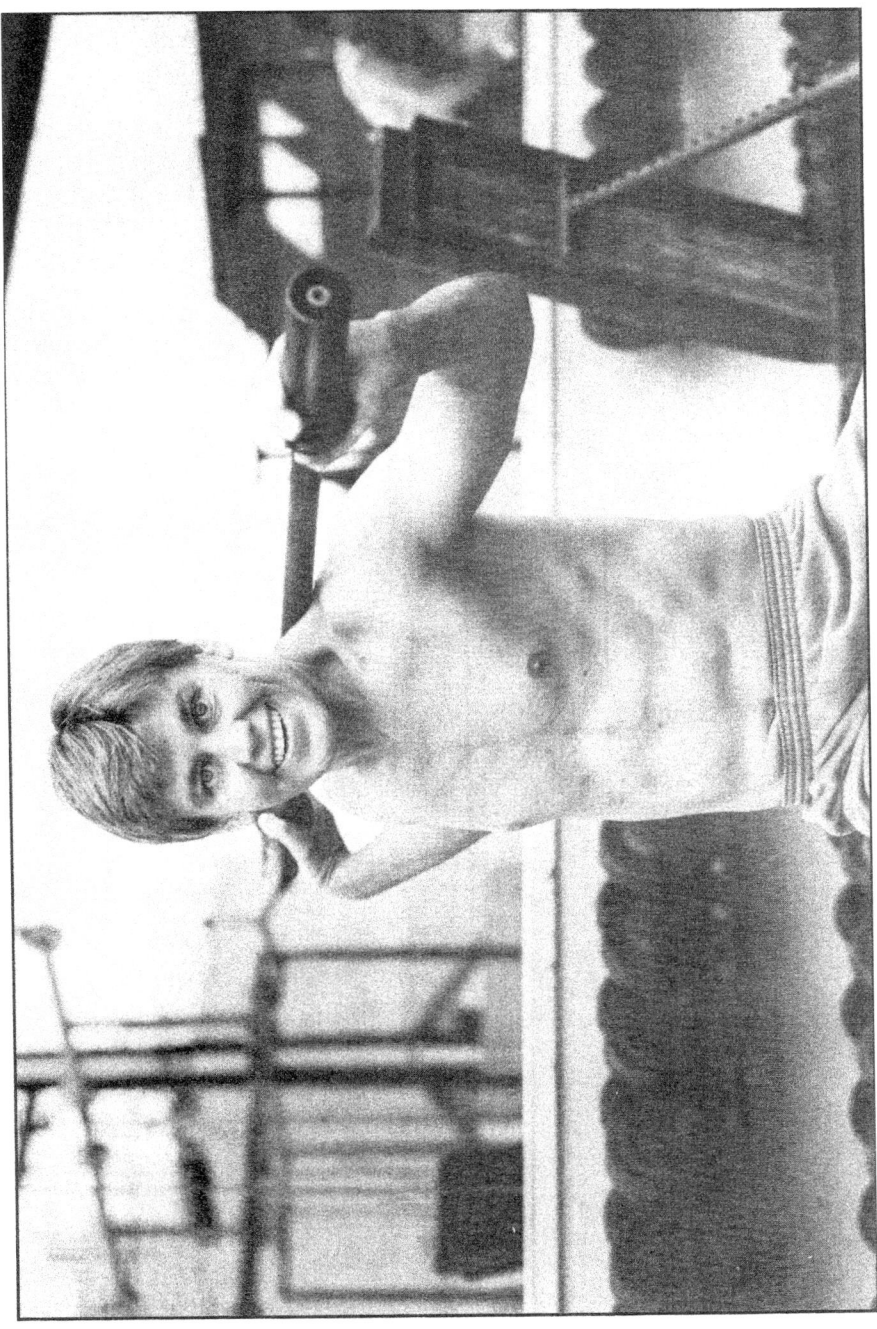

Trunk Twists With Empty Bar: This exercise works the entire abdominals. Trunk twists should be done with a high number of reps for best results.

Photo by Leon Bach at World Gym in Venice, California

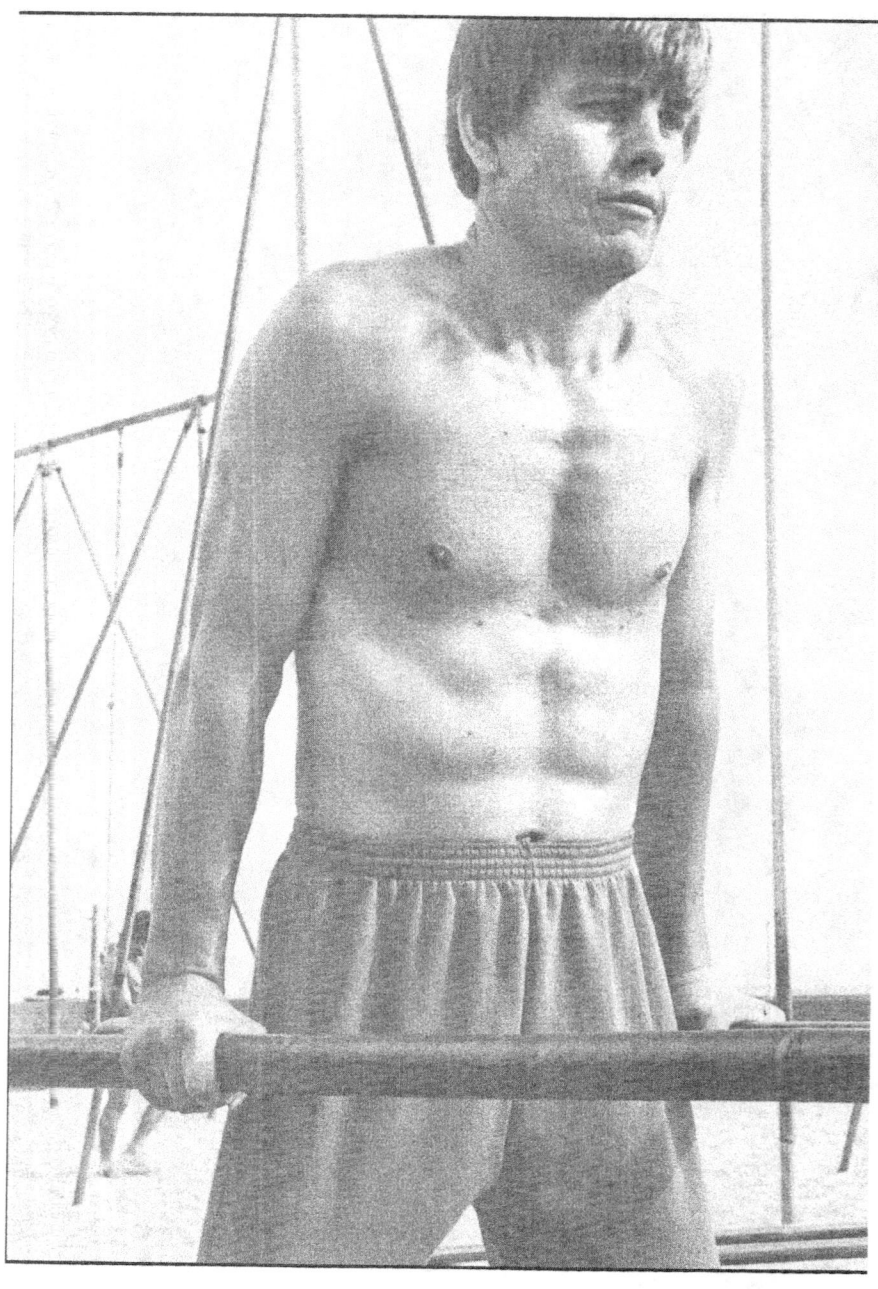

Dips are great for the Serratus and Intercostals. On this exercise go all the way up and all the way down. Do dips on the days you train your chest because dips are also great for the chest.

Photo by Leon Bach at World Gym in Venice, California

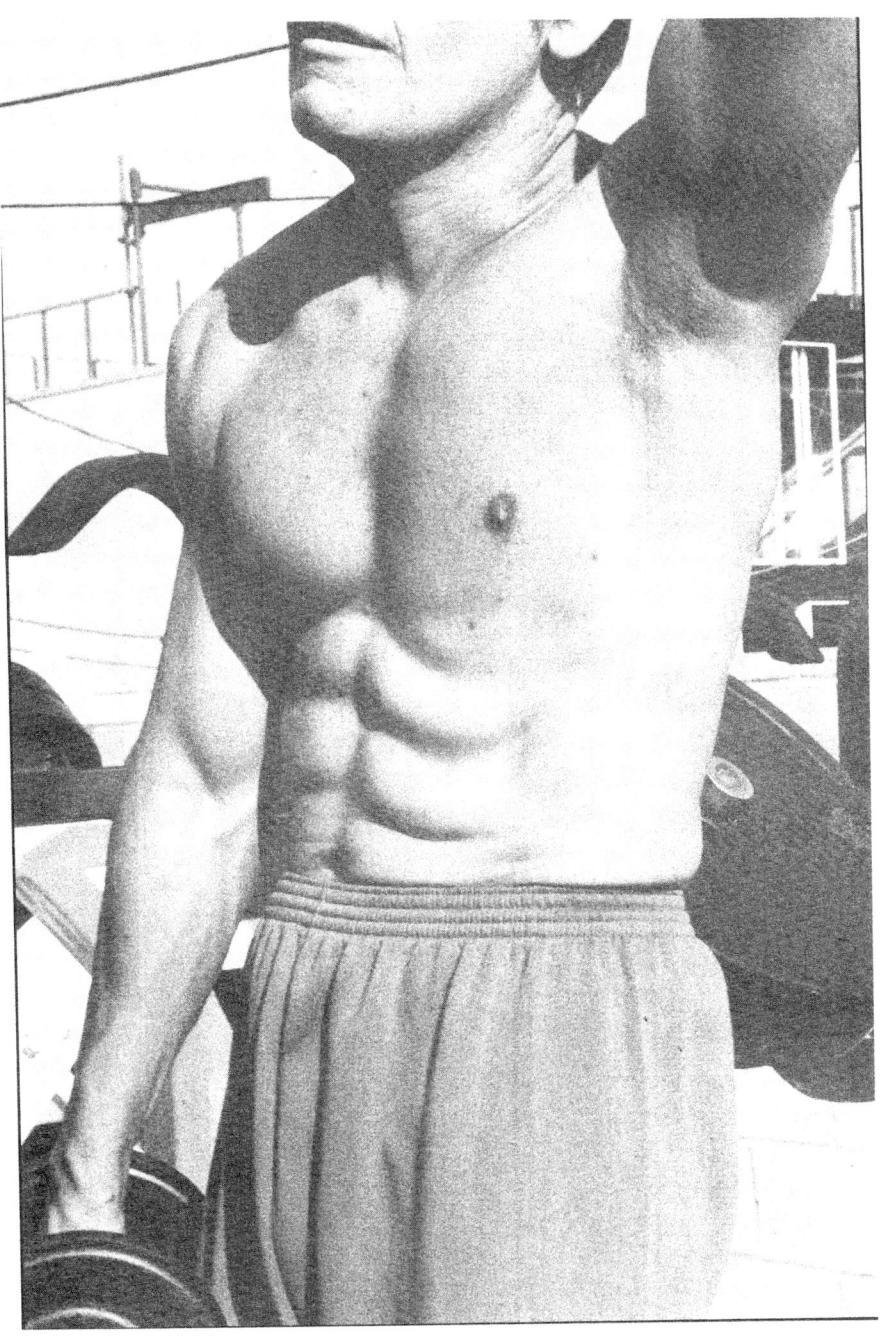

Side bends: When performing side bends always do high repetitions. Place one hand on head, hold dumbbell in other hand and rock back & forth.

Photo by Leon Bach at World Gym in Venice, California

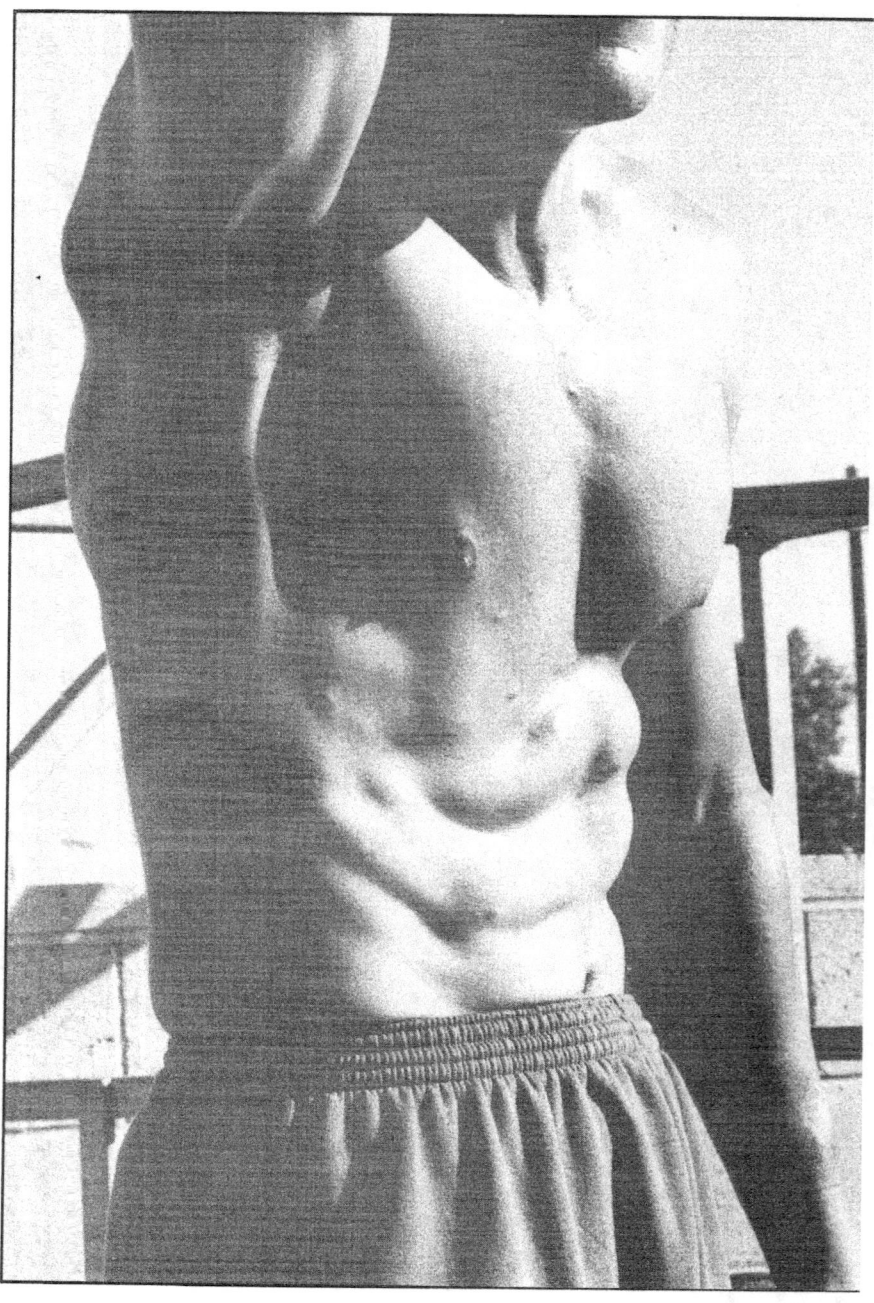

Side Bends: Close up photo showing Serratus and Intercostals. Do a high number of reps on the exercise.

Photo by Leon Bach at World Gym in Venice, California

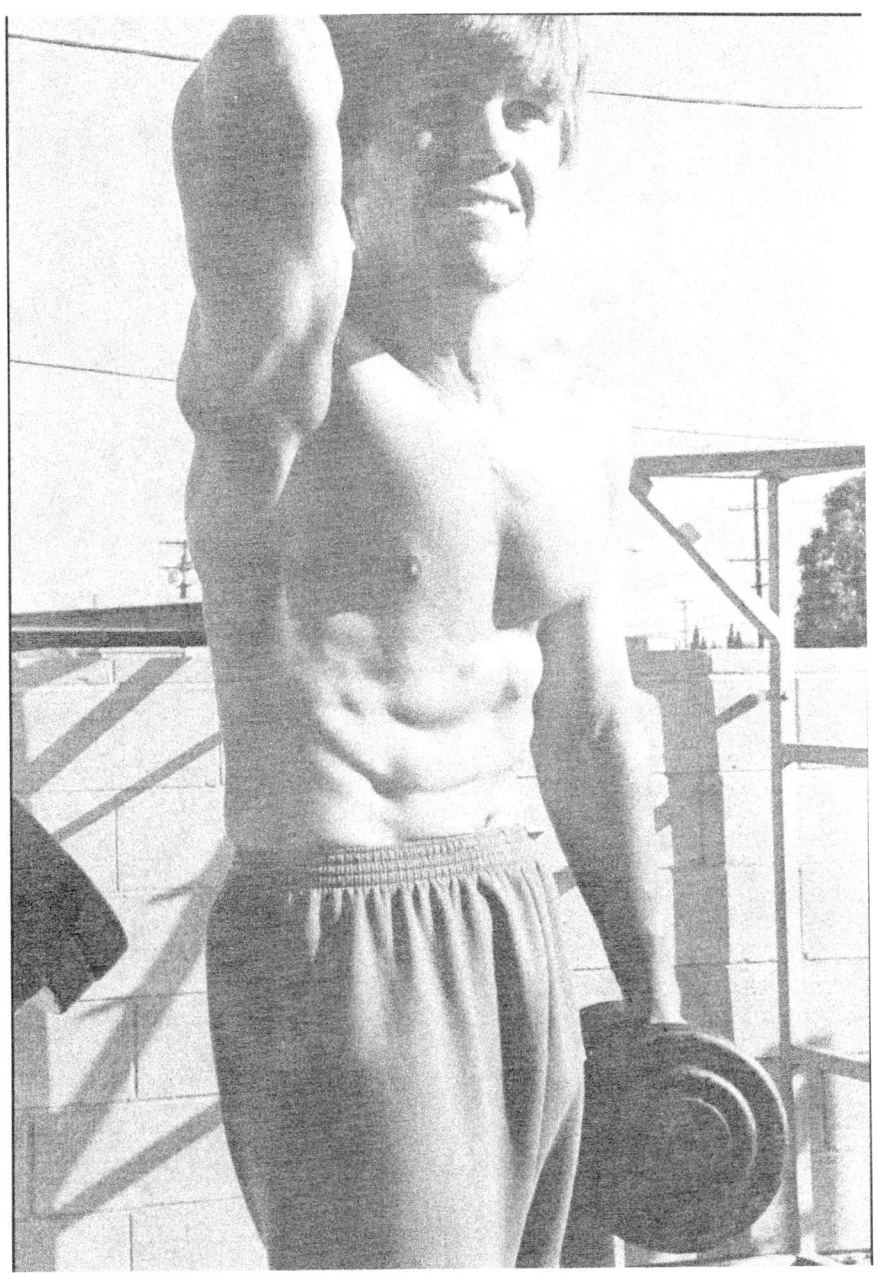

Side bends are great for the Serratus, Intercostal and Oblique Muscles. Use a dumbbell that is not too heavy for this exercise. Use good form.

Photo by Leon Bach at World Gym in Venice, California

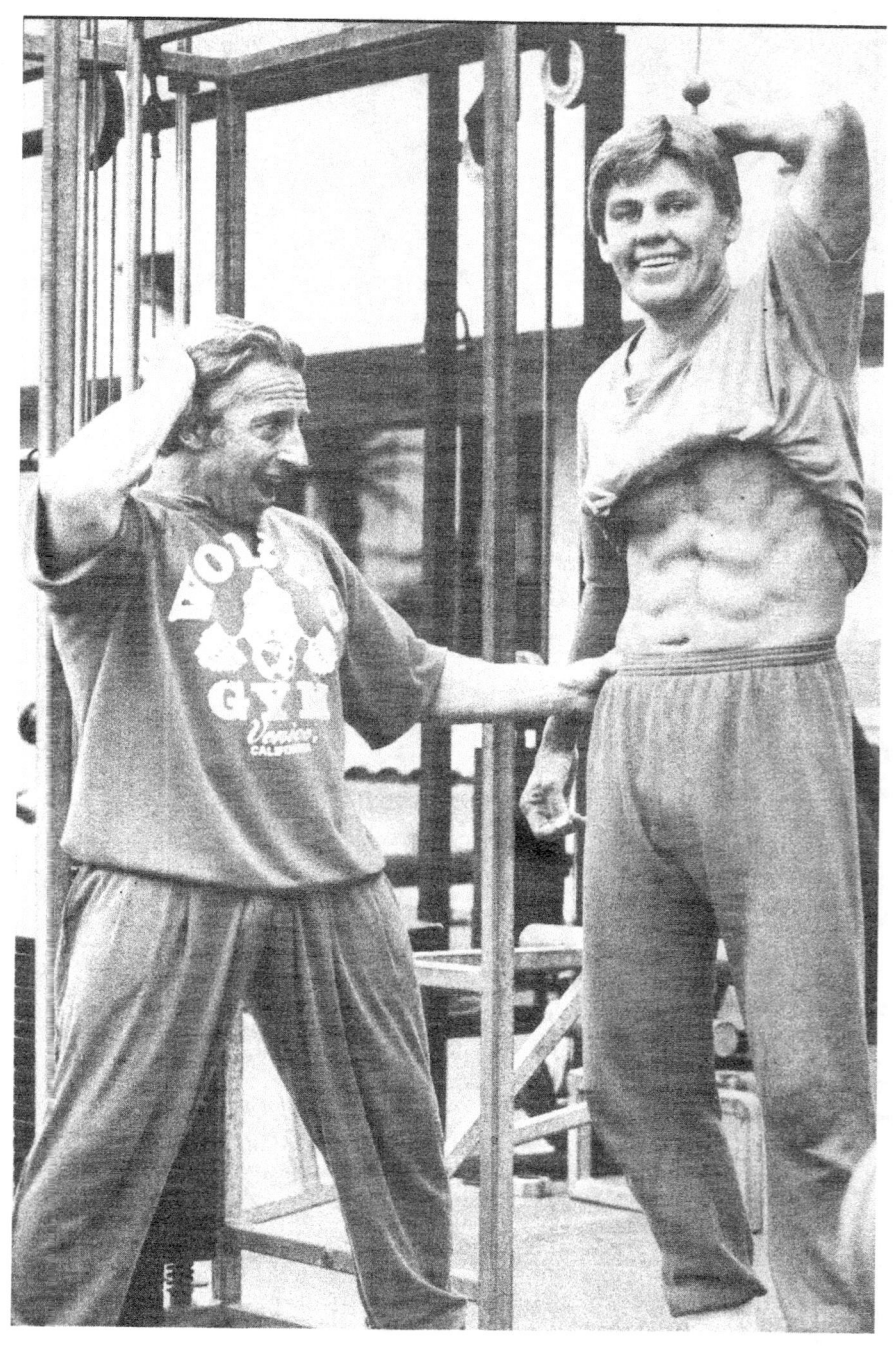

I'm pictured with Eddie Giuliani

Photo by Leon Bach at World Gym in Venice, California

DEVELOPING PRIZE WINNING ABDOMINALS

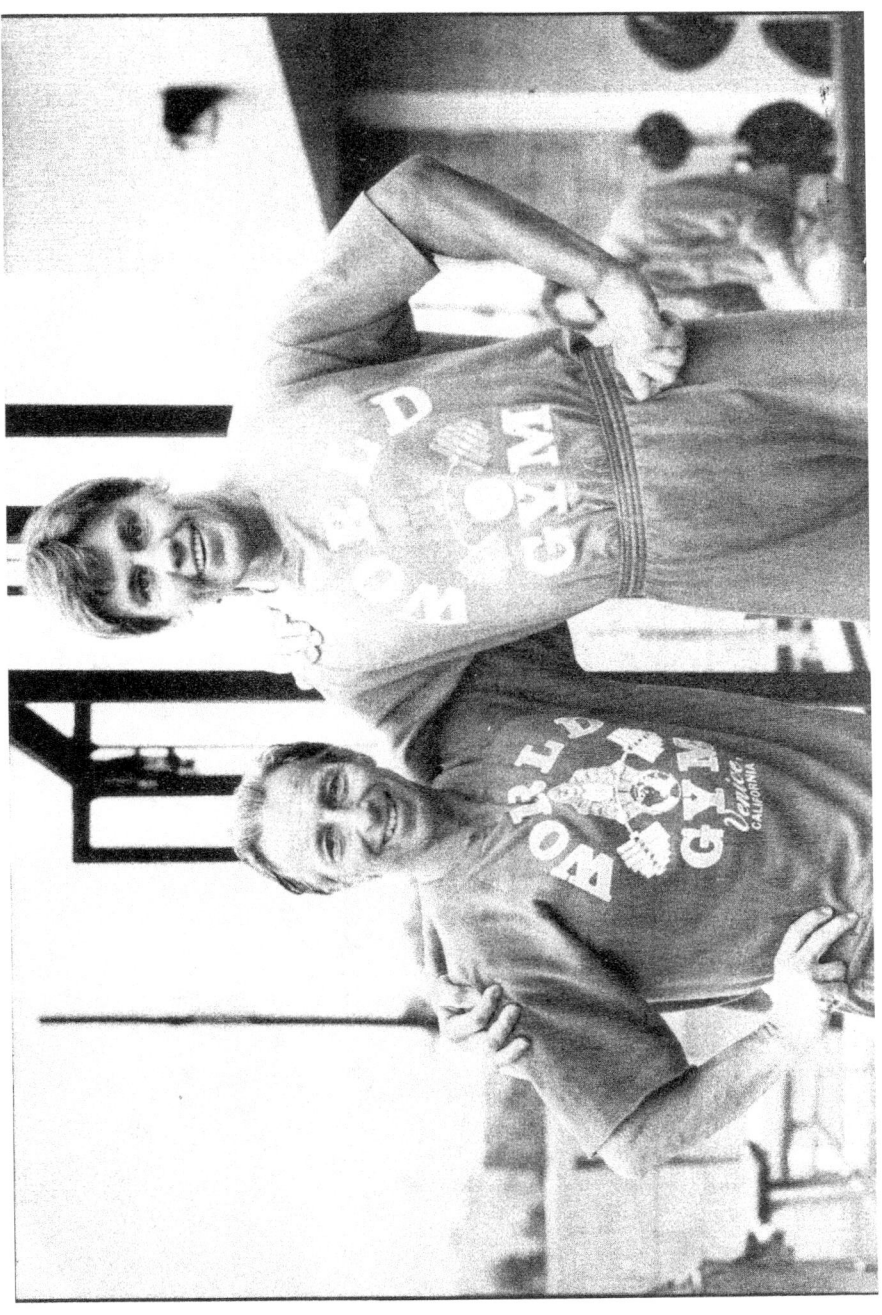

Eddie and I pose for a photo before a workout.

Photo by Leon Bach at World Gym in Venice, California

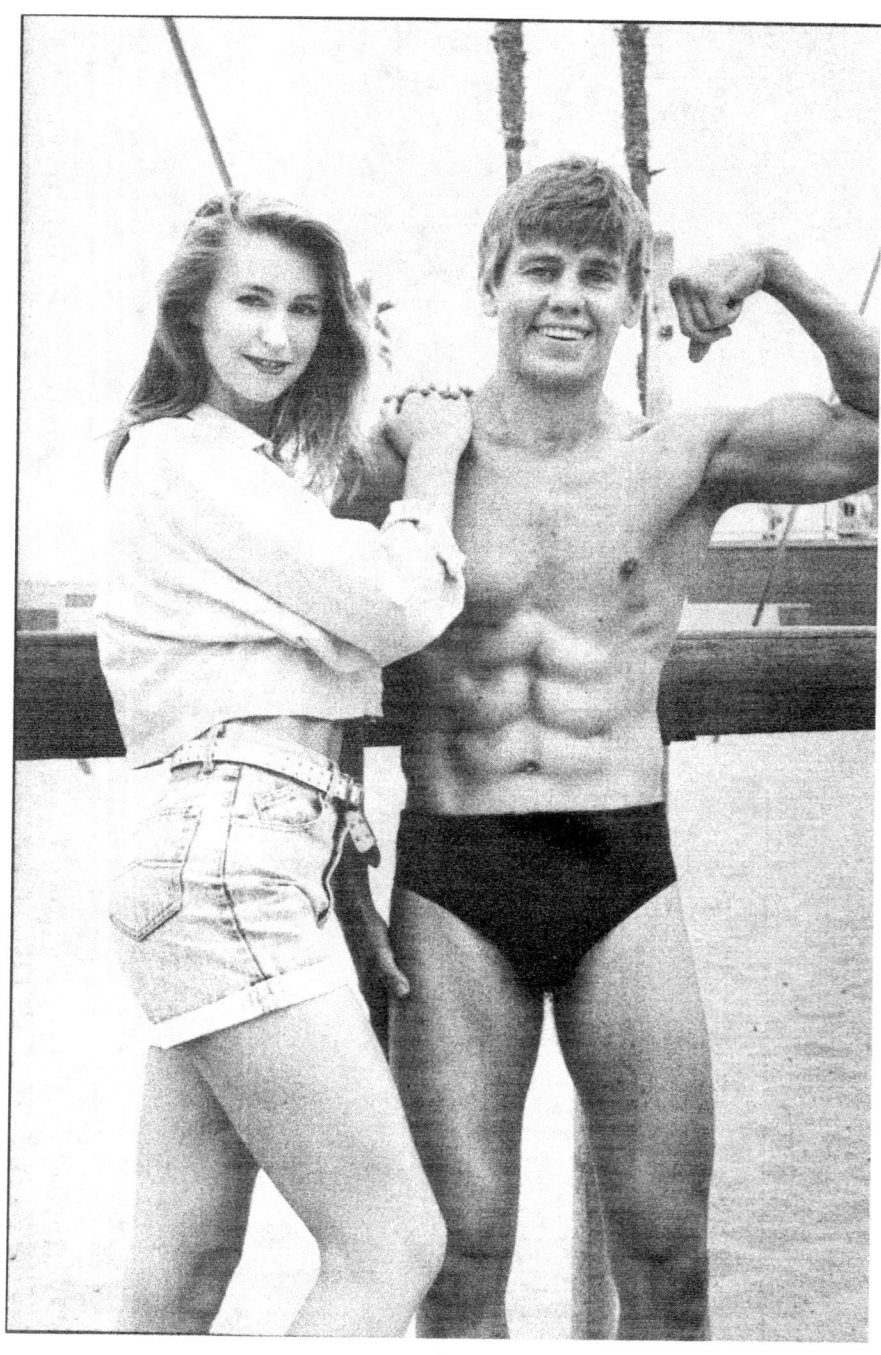

I am pictured with Faith Walker at Muscle Beach. Faith had a beautiful poster available through Ironman Magazine. The poster is called "Who's That Girl?".

Photo by Leon Bach in Venice, California

DEVELOPING PRIZE WINNING ABDOMINALS

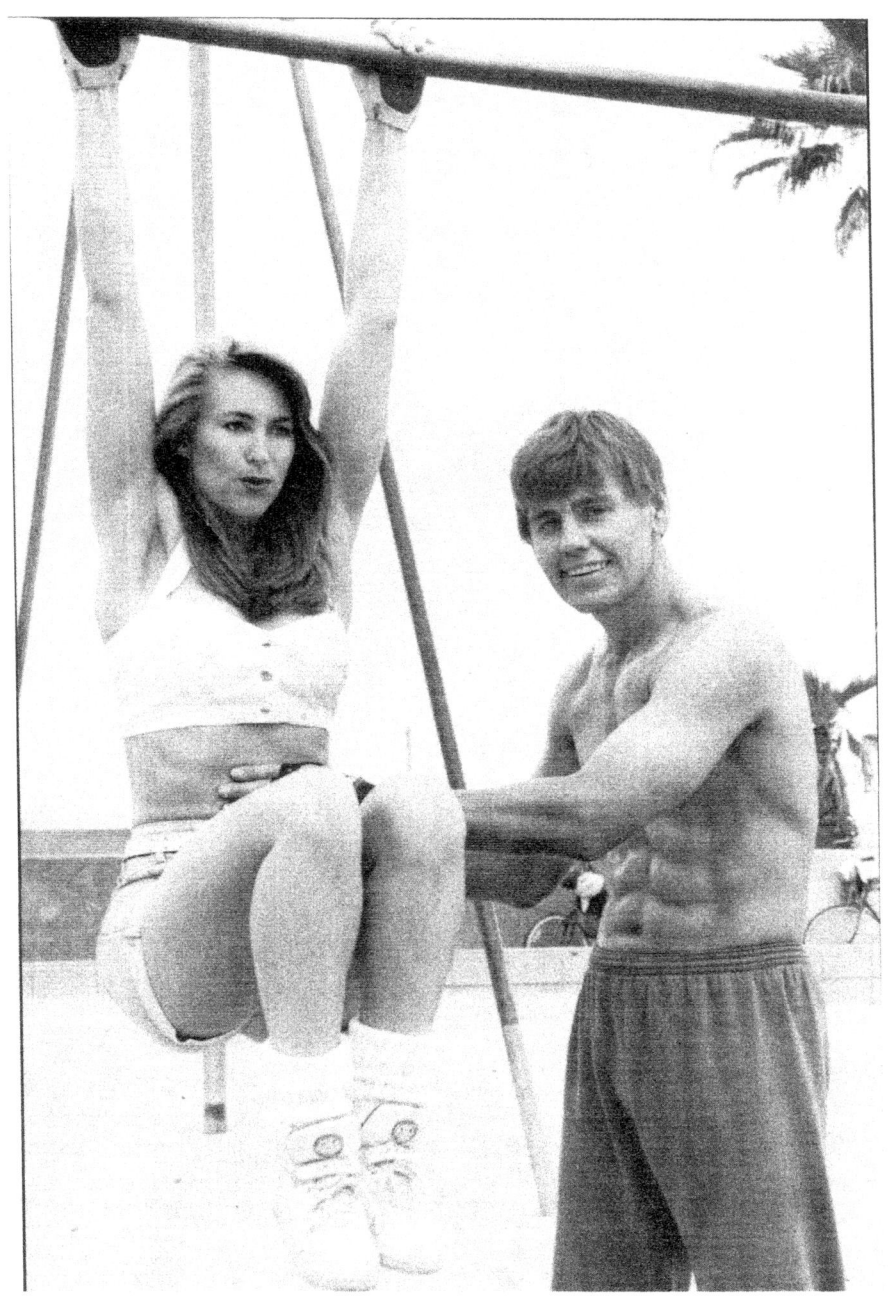

Guiding Faith Walker through a set of Hanging Leg Raises. Do a high number of reps on this exercise.

Photo by Leon Bach at World Gym in Venice, California

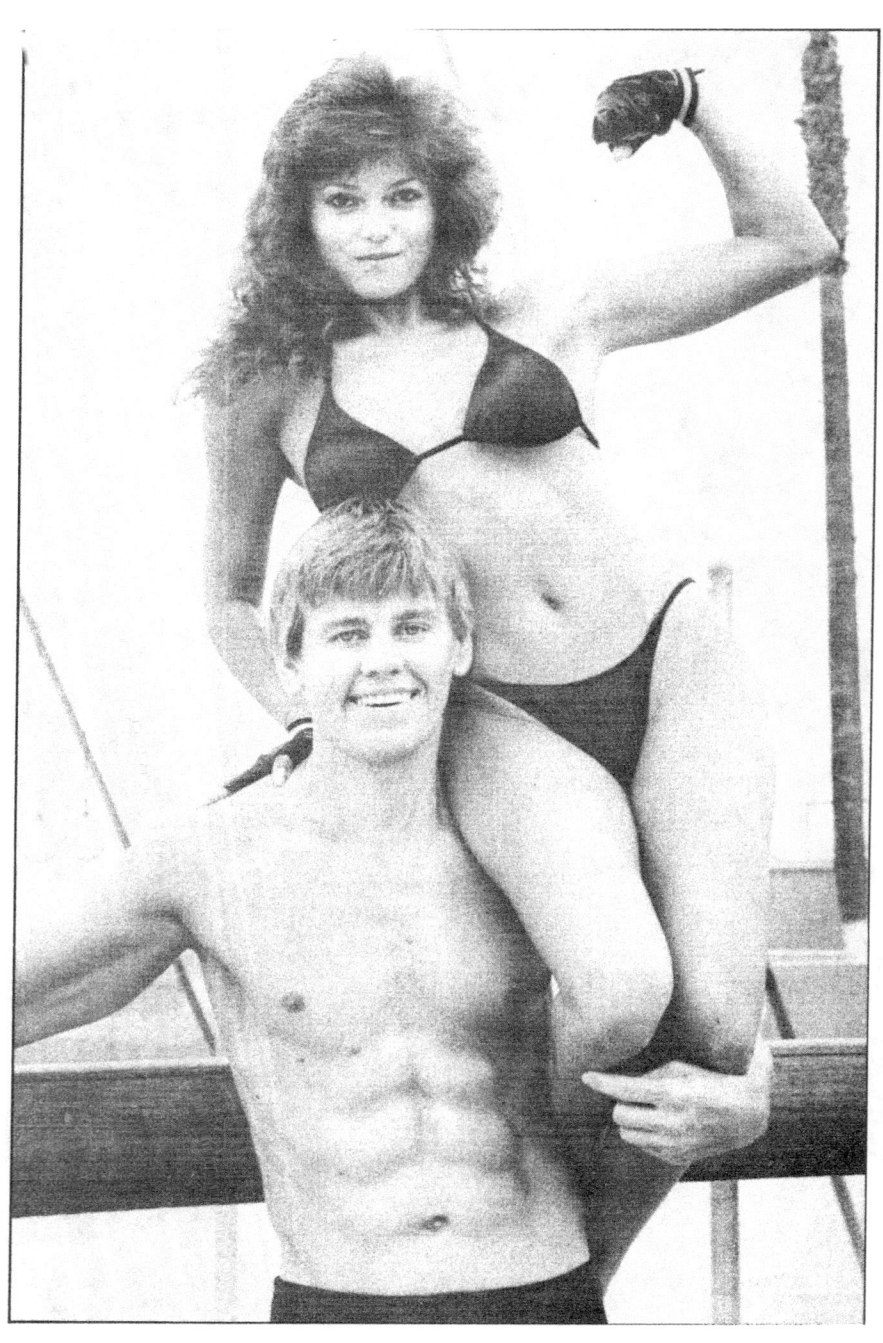

I am pictured with my friend Janet Hathaway, a top swim suit model.

Photo by Leon Bach, Muscle Beach, Venice, California.

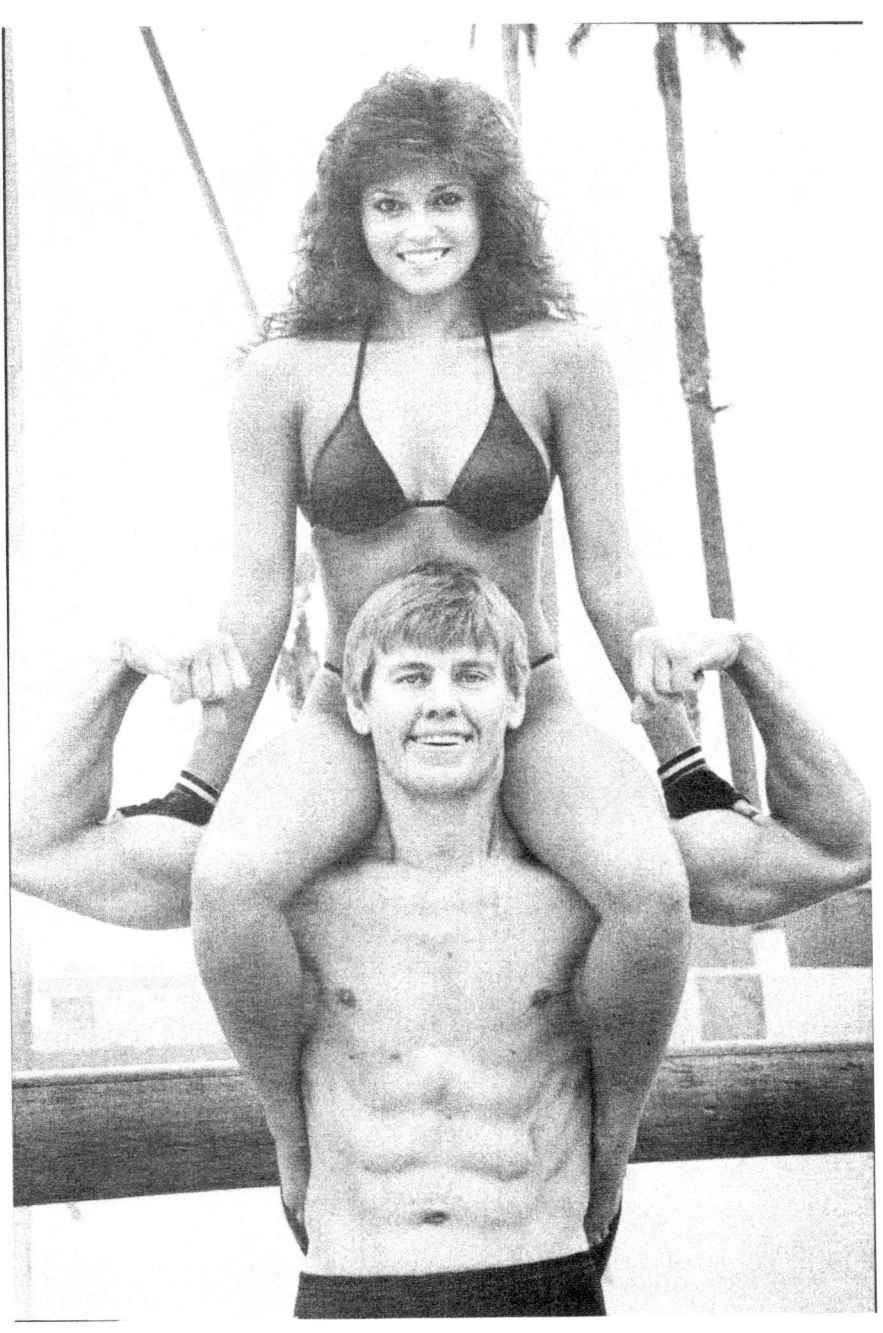

I am with my friend Janet Hathaway, a top swim suit model. This picture was taken at Muscle Beach in Venice, California

Photo by Leon Bach

by DOUG BROLUS

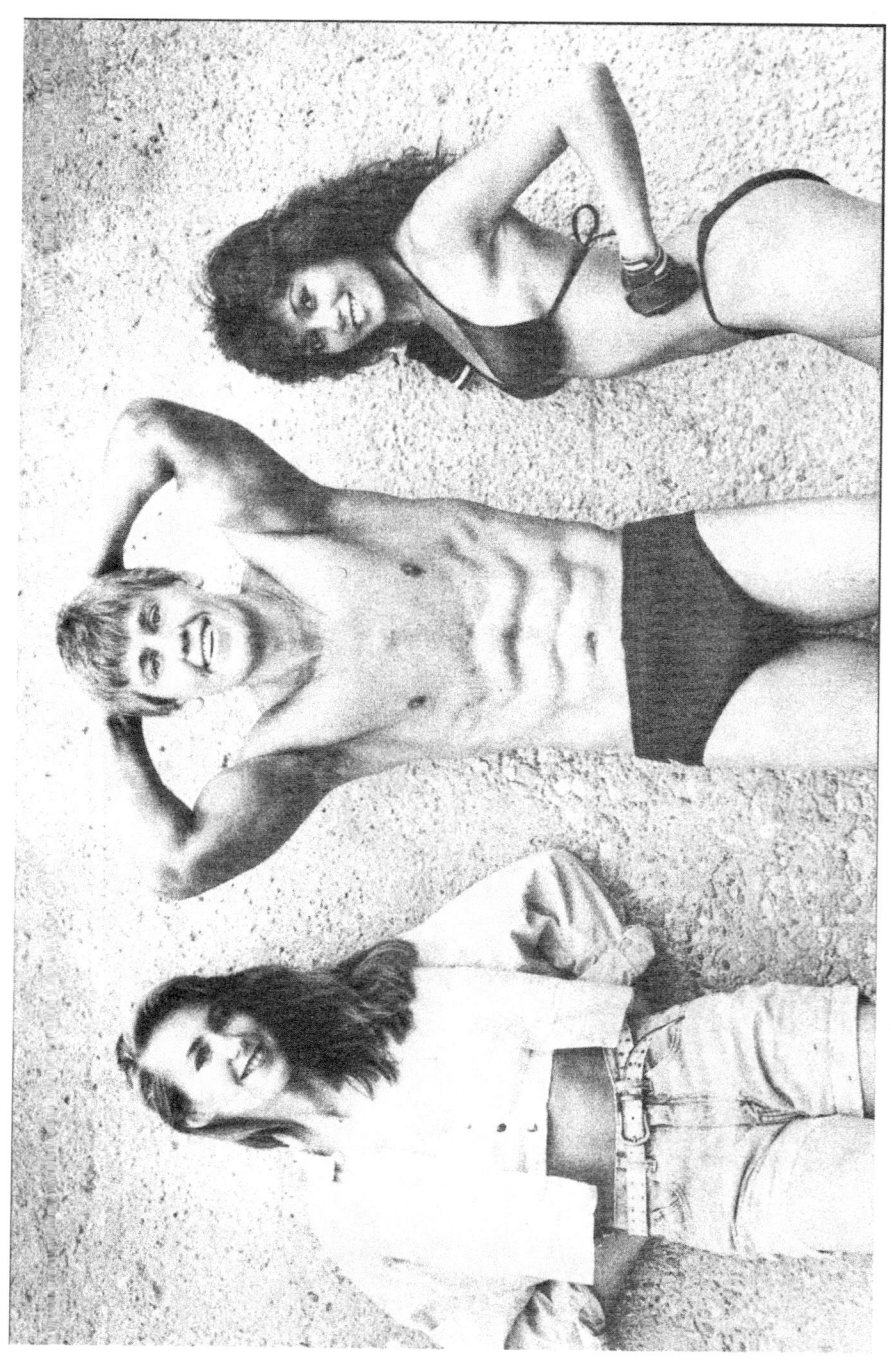

I'm pictured with Faith Walker and Swim Suit Model Janet Hathaway at Muscle Beach

Photo by Leon Bach at World Gym in Venice, California

DEVELOPING PRIZE WINNING ABDOMINALS

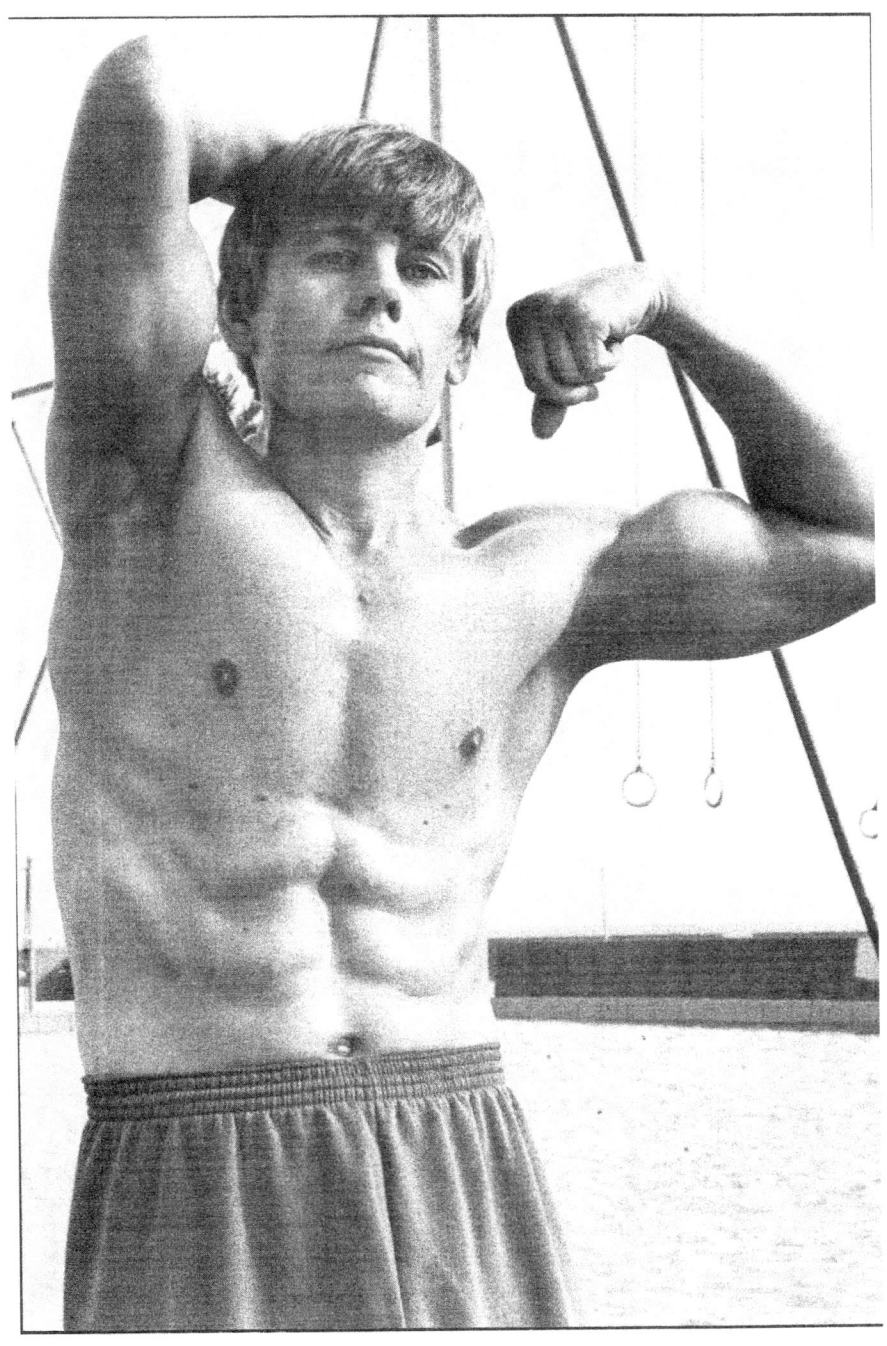

Early evening on Muscle Beach, Venice, California

Photo by Leon Bach

by DOUG BROLUS

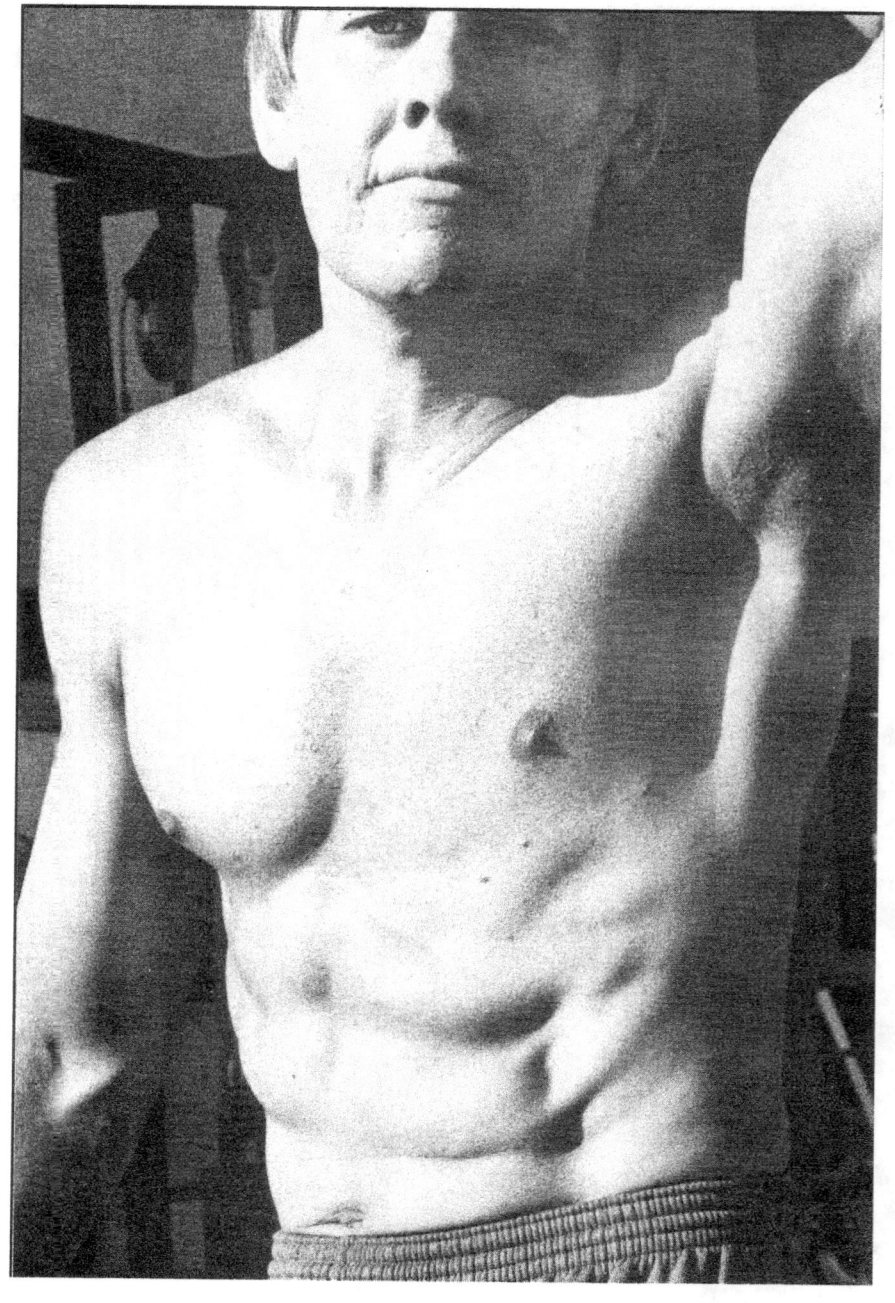

This photo shows the Serratus and Intercostal Muscles. It takes a lot of hard work to bring the abs out but it is worth it.

Photo by Leon Bach at World Gym in Venice, California

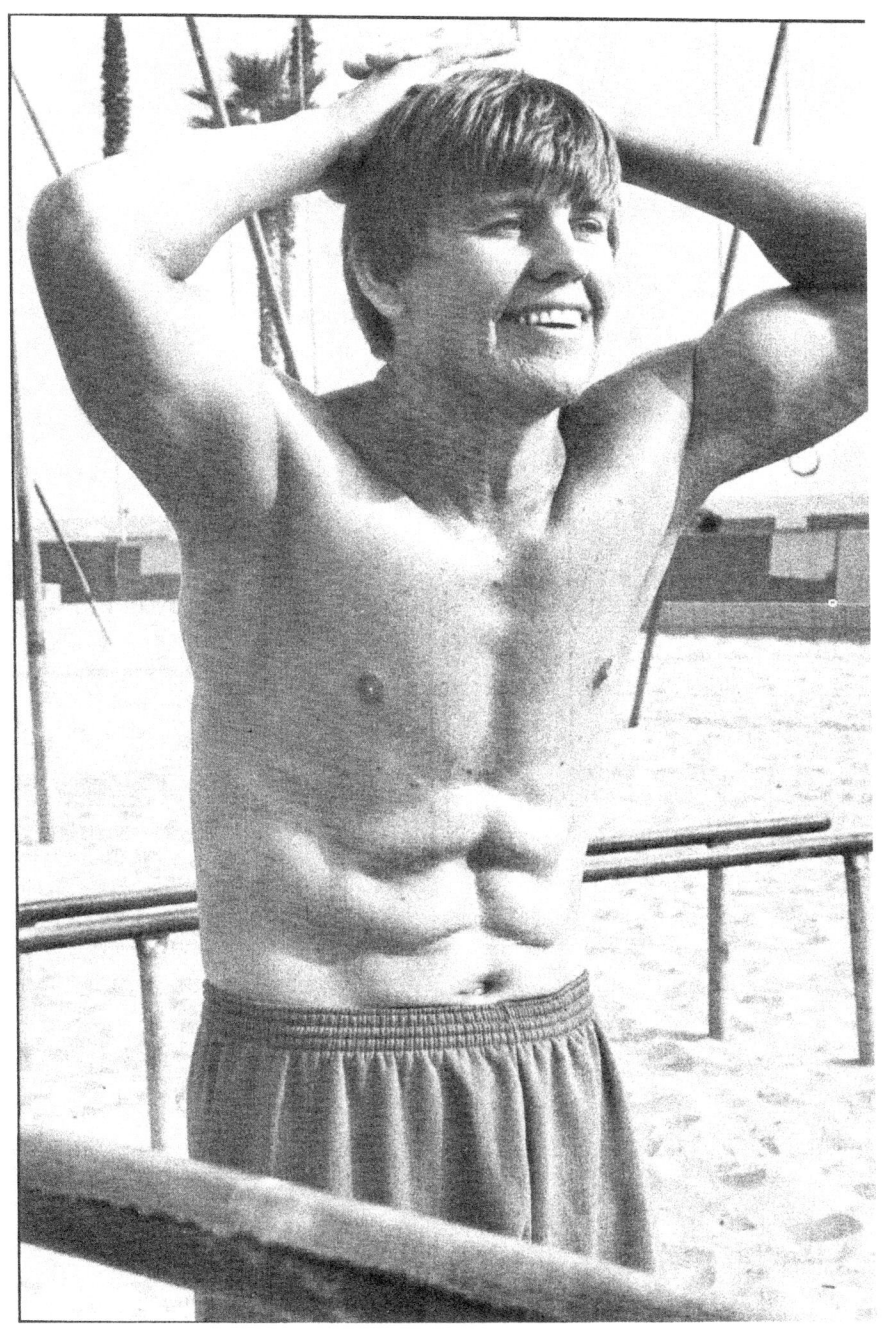

Muscle Beach in the early evening, Venice, California

Photo by Leon Bach

by **DOUG BROLUS**

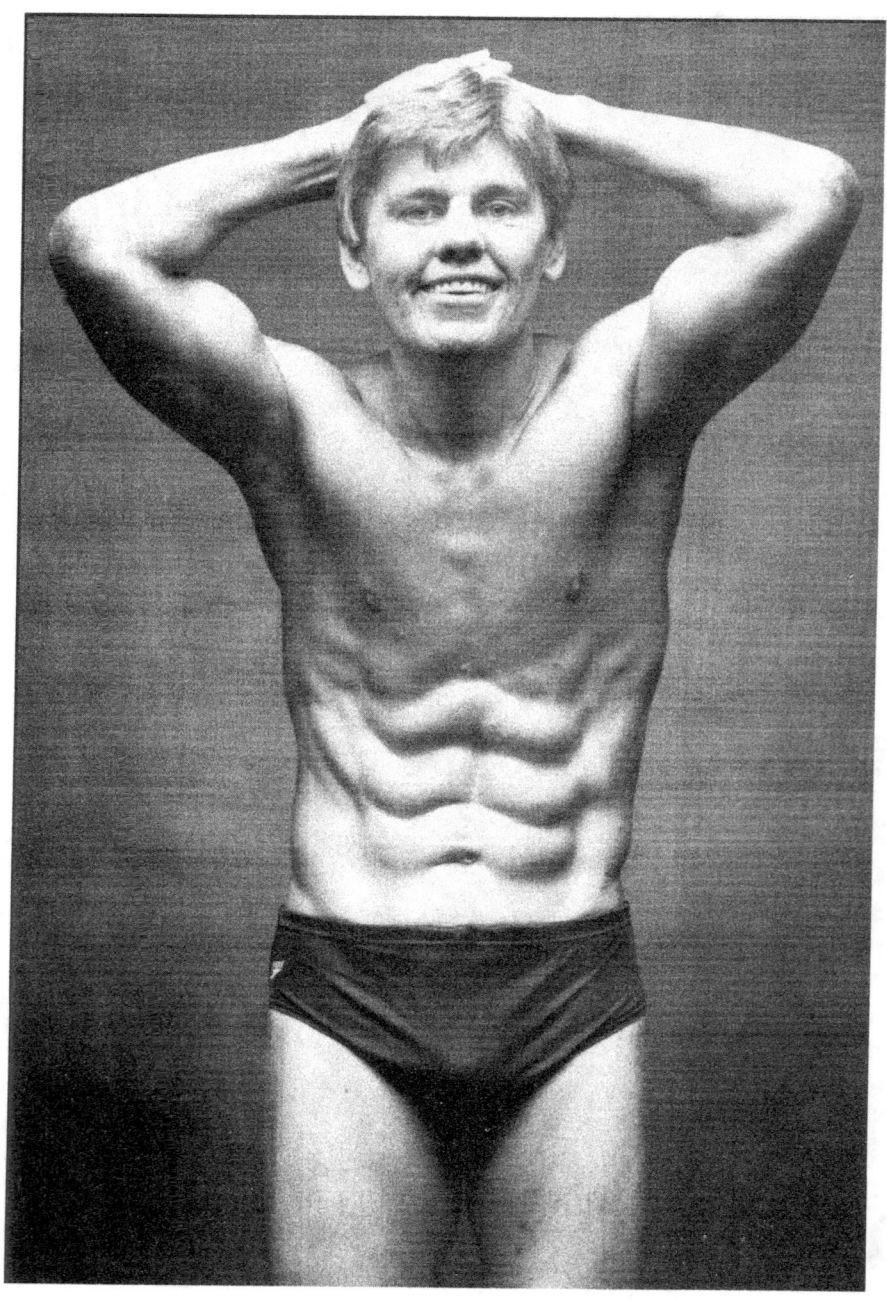

This picture shows the Rectus Abdominals.

Photo by Dave Siegle, Hollywood, California

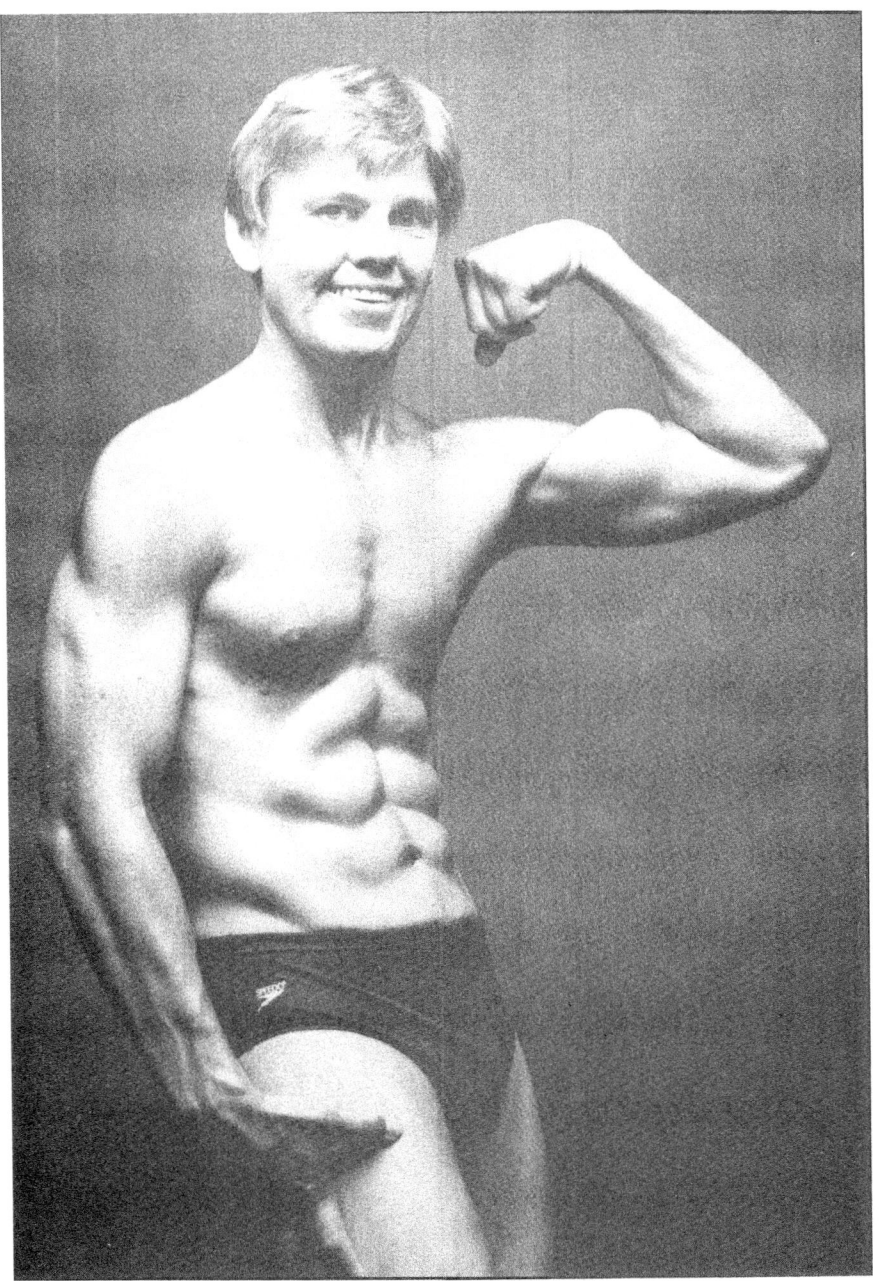

This picture shows the abs and upper body flexed. Keep the body in proportion. Do not train one muscle group to out-do the other parts. Balance is the key.

Photo by Dave Siegle, Hollywood, California

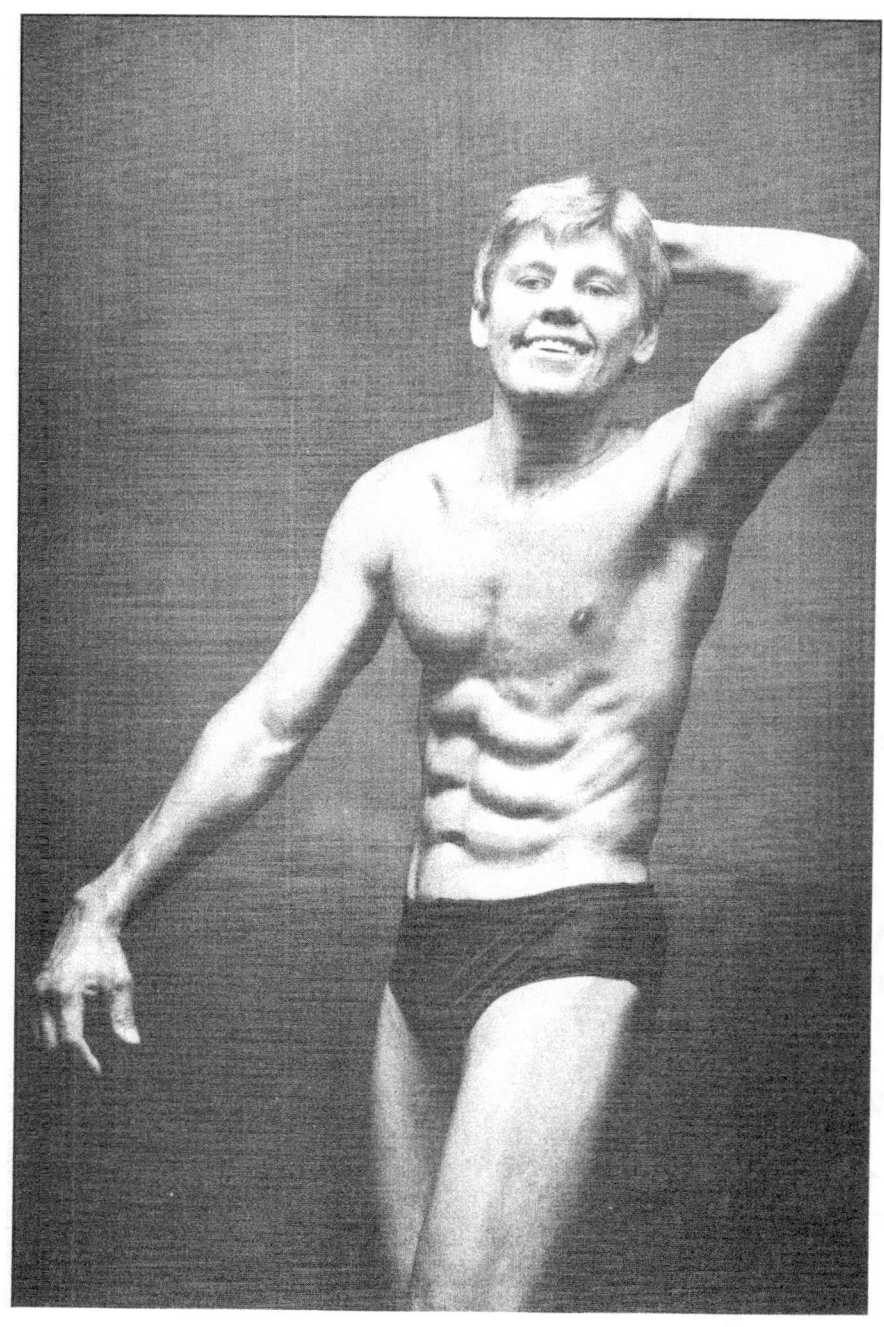

The photo shows the Serratus, Intercostals and Rectus Abdominals.

Photo by Dave Siegle, Hollywood, California

DEVELOPING PRIZE WINNING ABDOMINALS

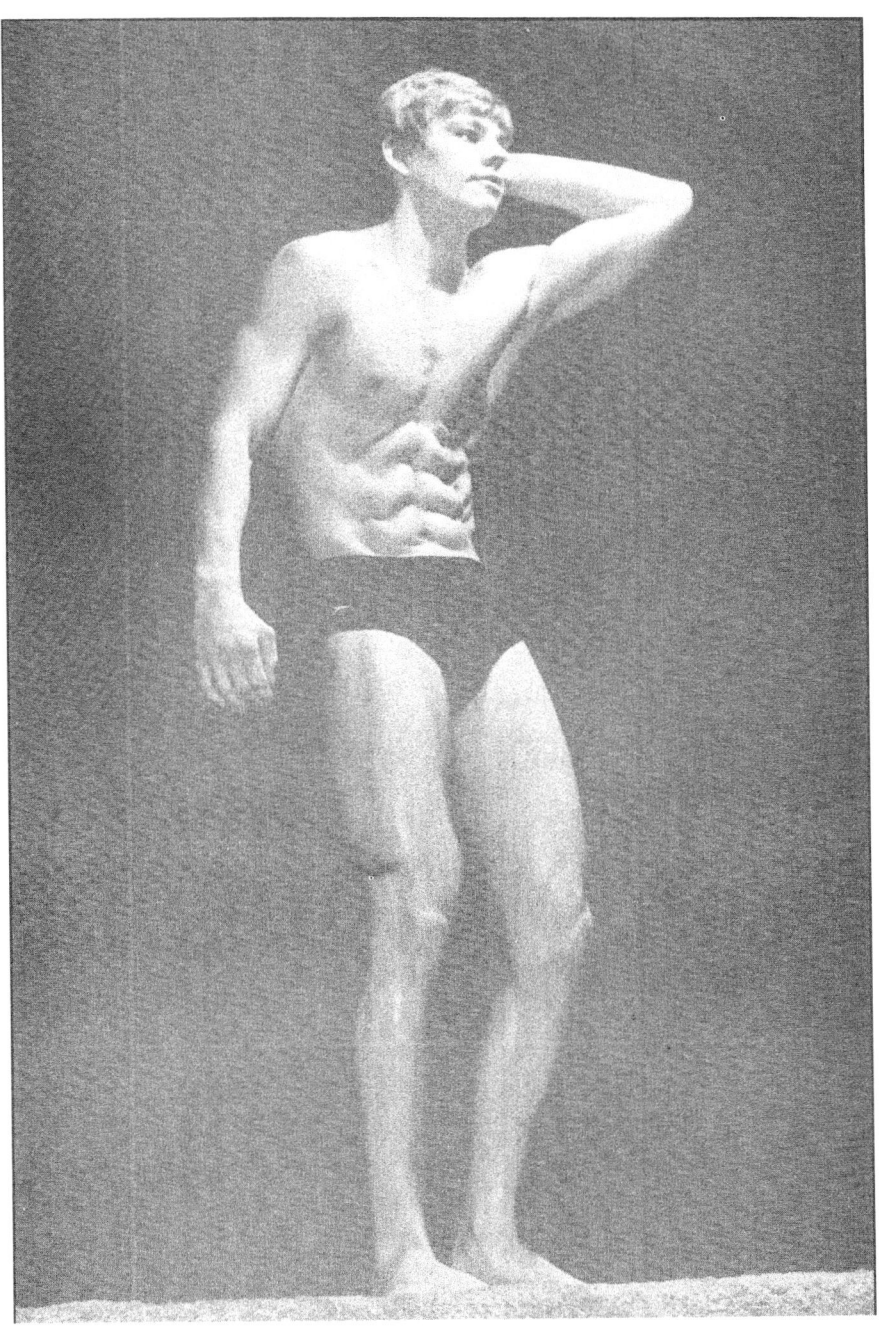

This is the Competition Look on Stage

Photo by Dan Hartner

by **DOUG BROLUS**

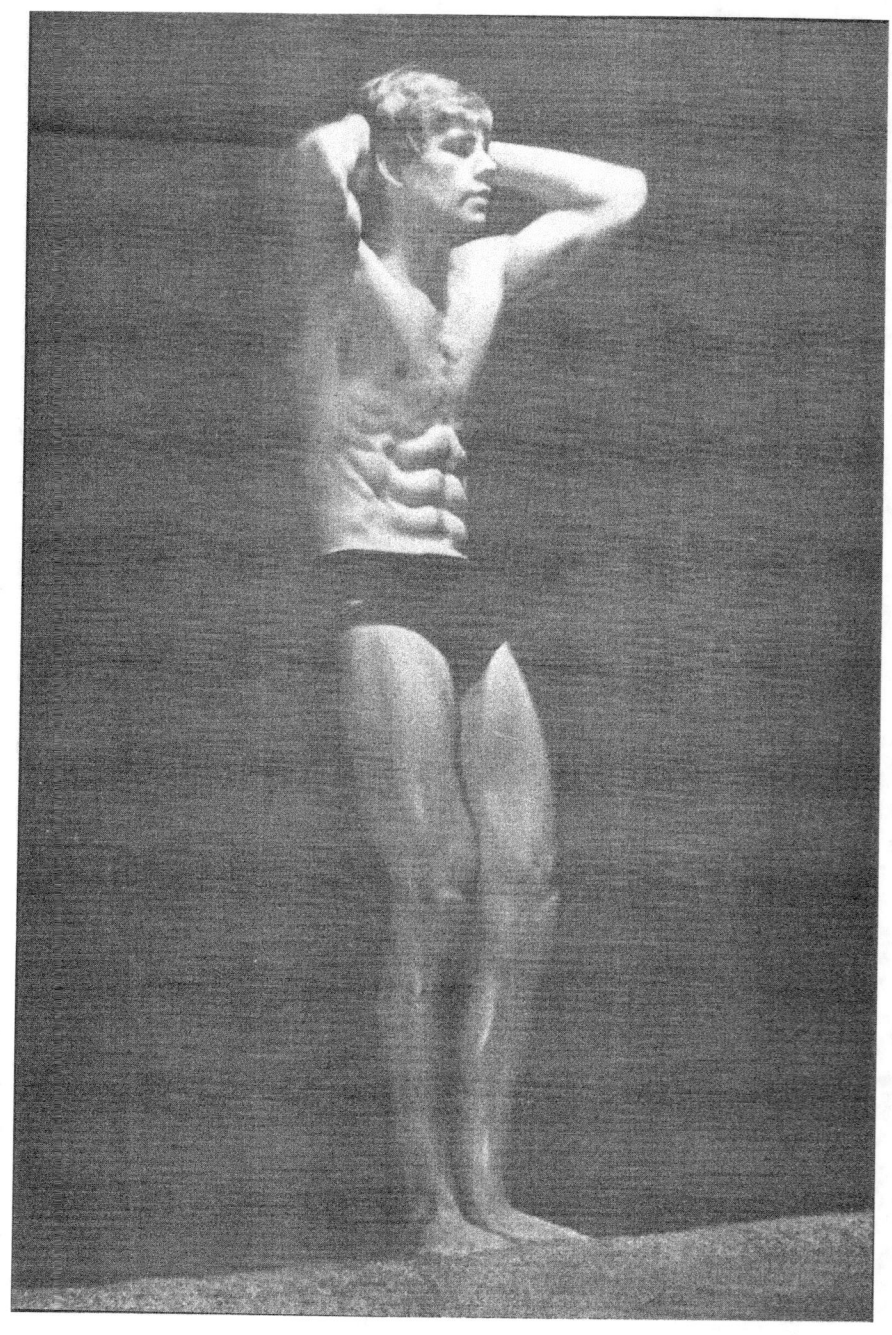

This is the Competition Look on Stage

Photo by Dan Hartner

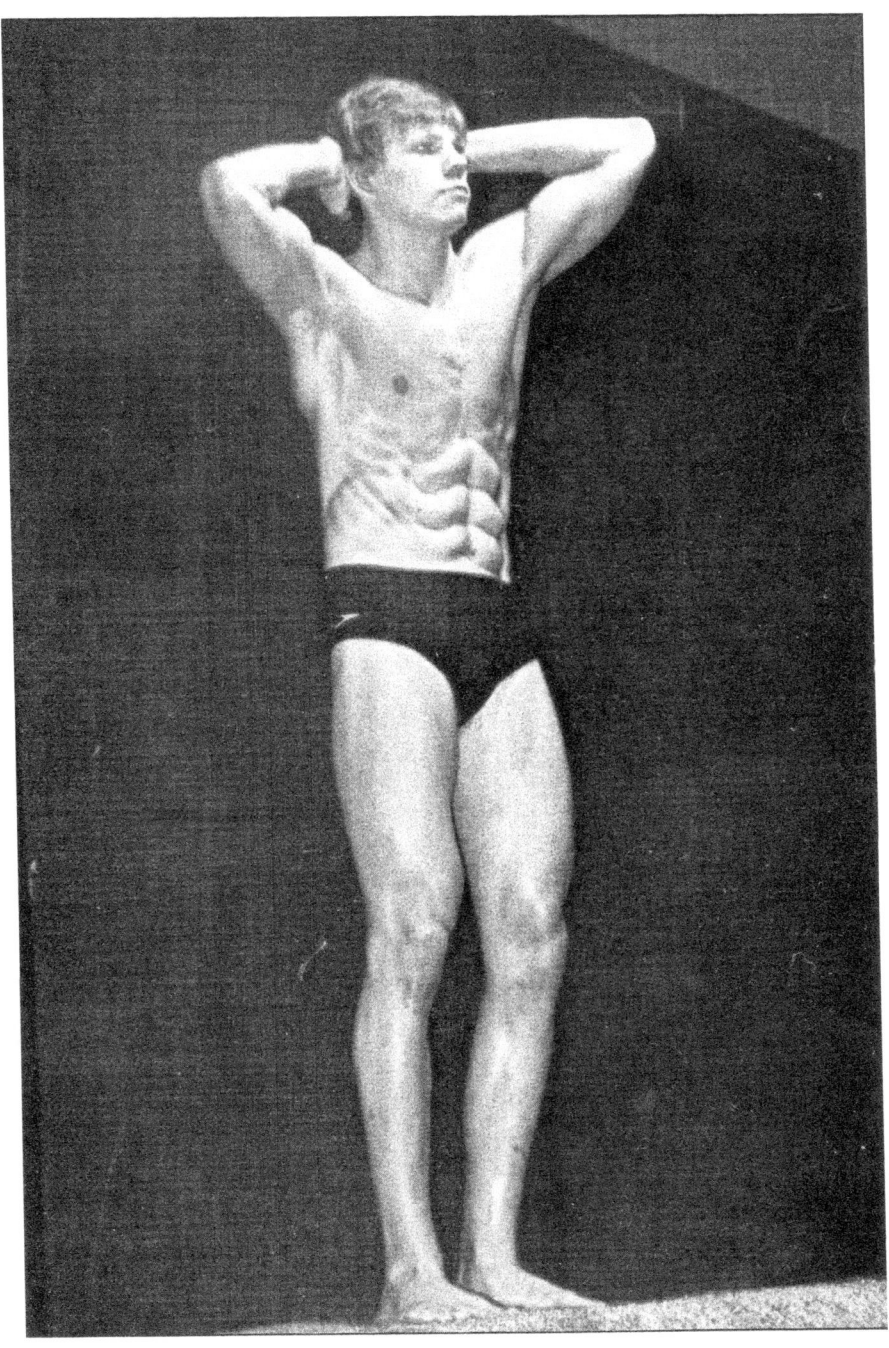

Here I am winning best abdominals. Competition Posing on stage.

Photo by Dan Hartner

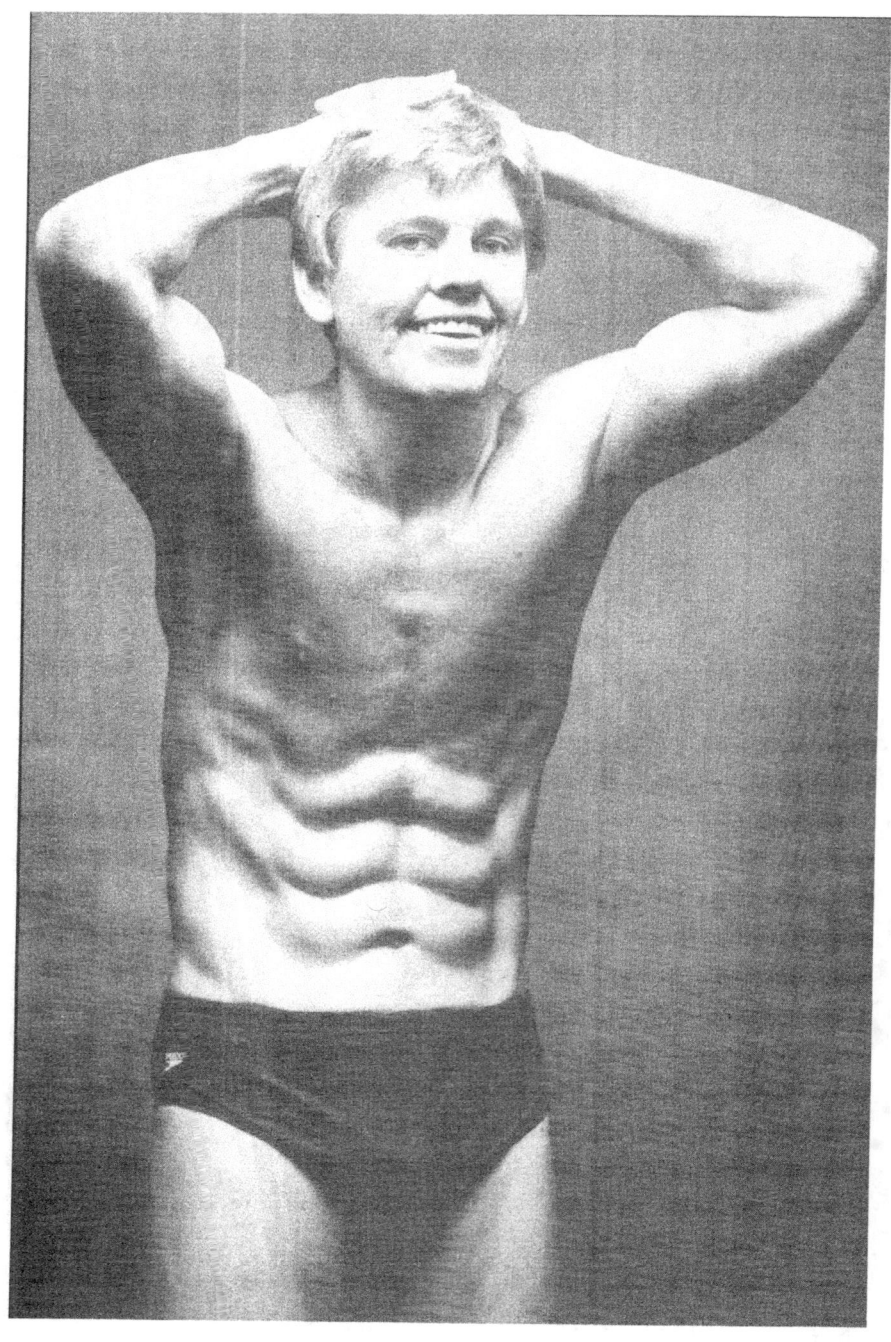

Photo by Dave Siegle, Hollywood, California

DEVELOPING PRIZE WINNING ABDOMINALS

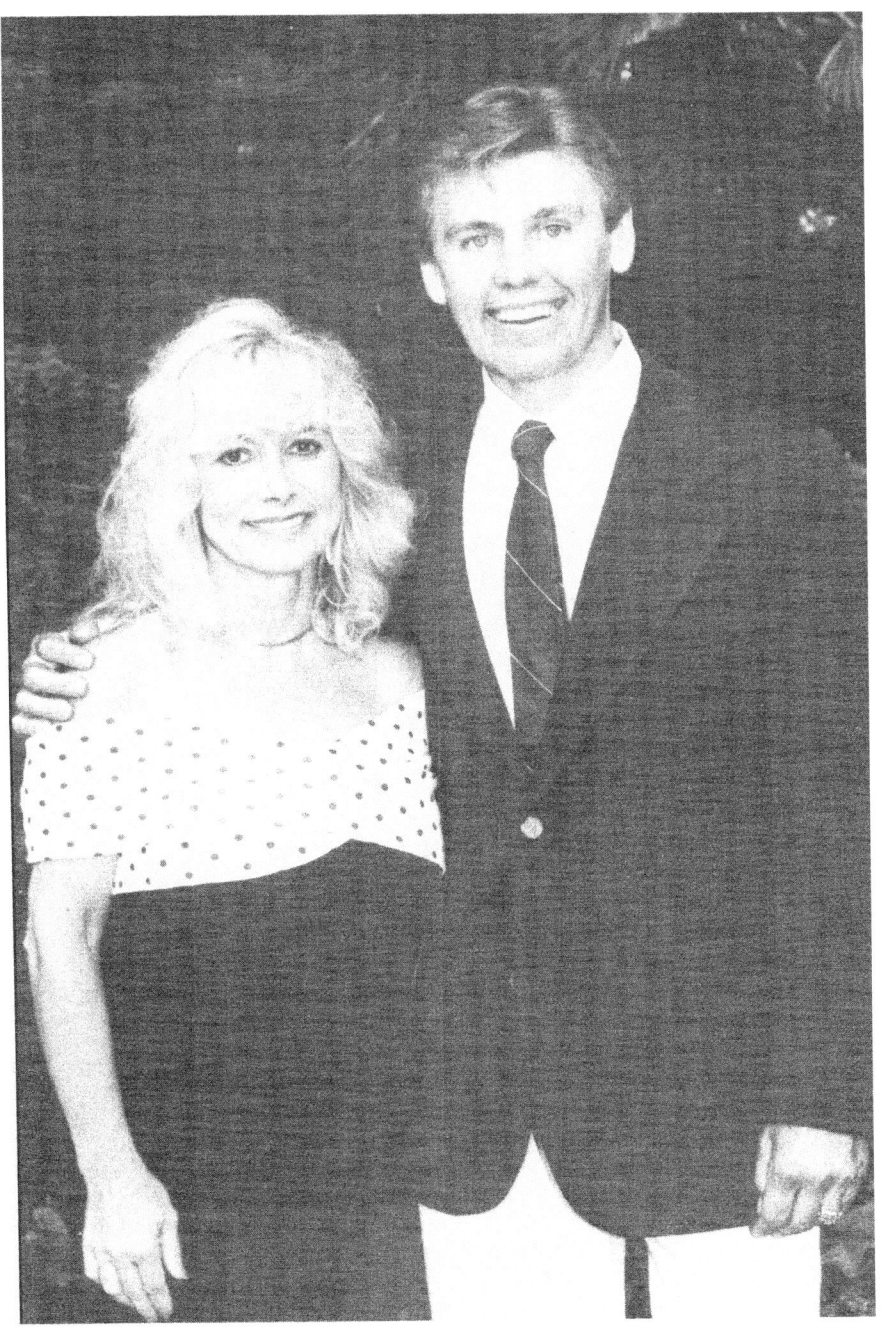

I'm pictured with Patricia Stephenson, my former publicist.

Photo by Dave Siegle

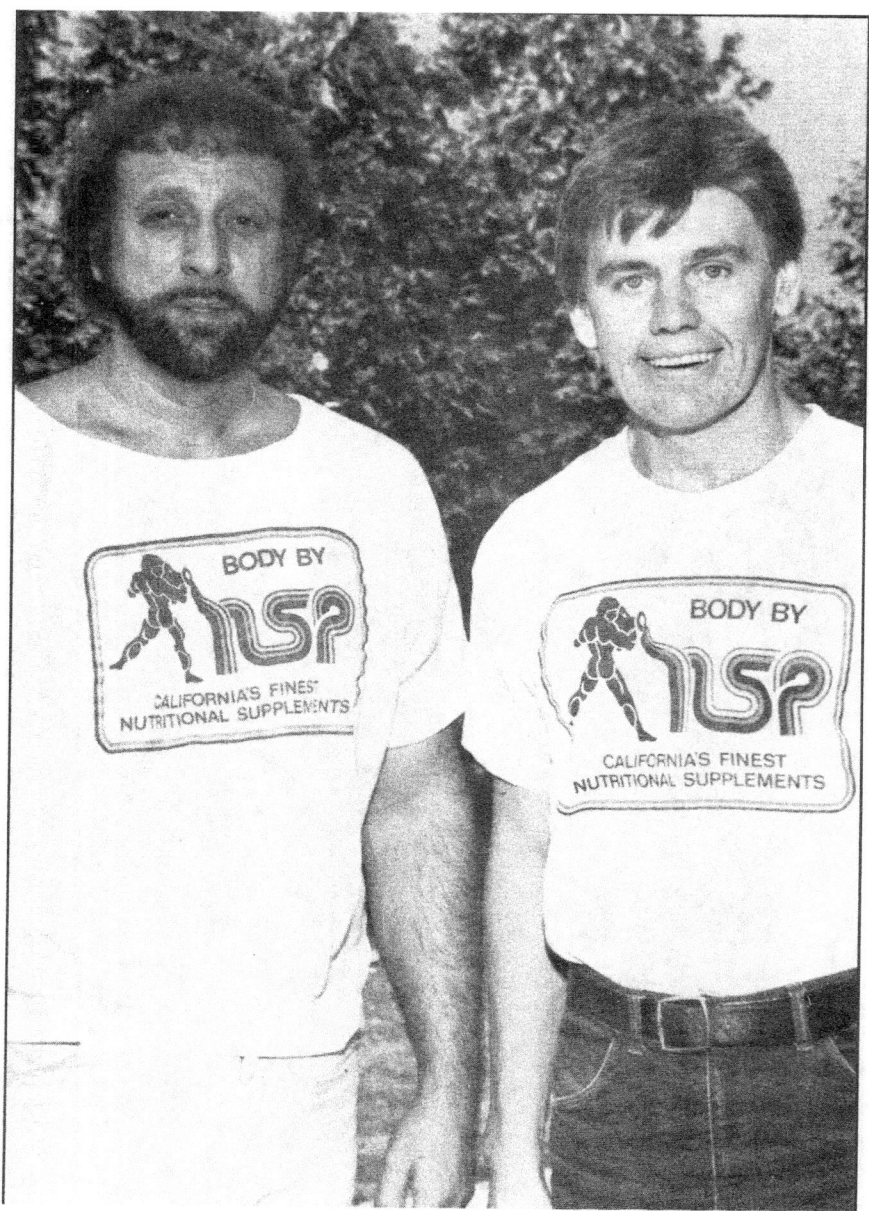

Nutritional Supplements

With Doug is Ron Kosloff, owner of Natural Source Products in Detroit, Michigan. I would like to thank Ron for all his help with my training and diet. If you are interested in any of the NSP products, call him at 1-313-372-1807 for a free catalogue and price list.

Photo by Tom Mobley

The diet you should follow is very high in protein and low in carbohydrates.

Proteins are a source of heat and energy to the body. They are essential for growth, the building of new tissue and repair of injuries or broken down tissues.

They form an integral part of the protoplasm of every cell. They are oxidized in the body, thus liberating heat. One gram of protein supplies 4 calories of heat.

The best proteins to eat are meat, fish, liver, eggs, turkey and chicken. These foods have all the complete amino acids to make each one of them a complete protein.

Carbohydrates are fruits, starches and vegetables and you can lose weight if you don't over do them. When you eat carbohydrates the body breaks them down for energy and if you consume too much carbohydrate you will not lose weight because your body has to draw from the fat stores for a person to lose weight. Your body will use carbohydrates for energy before it uses fats for energy, so don't eat too much of them. Eat just enough carbohydrates for energy, and when that is burned up with exercise, your body will start drawing from your fat stores for energy and you will begin to lose weight - as simple as that.

Balanced Diet for Super Abs

Breakfast
hot cereal
1 banana
apple juice and water
2 slices of whole wheat bread
1000 mg vitamin C
amino acids

Lunch
tuna fish mixed with a half of green pepper with Miracle Whip salad dressing
1 banana
1 apple
1 slice of whole wheat bread
1 B complex amino acids/water

Dinner
Half pound of fish
broccoli
1 banana
1 slice of bread
apple juice, 1000 mg vitamin C Amino acids

You can take larger amounts of vitamin B complex and vitamin C because these are water soluble and the body will not store them.

B complex helps appetite and is necessary for carbohydrate metabolism. Vitamin C helps build connective tissue in the body and strengthens muscle tissue.

Total Protein

One hundred and thirty-two grams (132 grams) protein.

Total Carbohydrates

One hundred and twenty grams (120 grams) carbohydrates

This diet is very healthy and can help you lose the weight you want to lose if you follow the foods listed and do the waist exercises.

Supplements You Should Take

Vitamin/Mineral tablet
B-complex
Vitamin C - 2000 milligrams
Vitamin E

You can take larger amounts of vitamin B-Complex and vitamin C because these are water soluble and body will not store them.

The vitamins that you don't want to overdo are A, D, E. These are fat soluble and store in the body.

Vitamins act principally as regulators of metabolic processes and play a role in energy transformation, usually acting as coenzymes in enzymatic systems.

Vitamin Action

A and D help growth
B-Complex helps appetite and is necessary for carbohydrate metabolism.
Vitamin C helps build connective tissue in the body and
strengthens muscle tissue.
Vitamin E will help endurance.

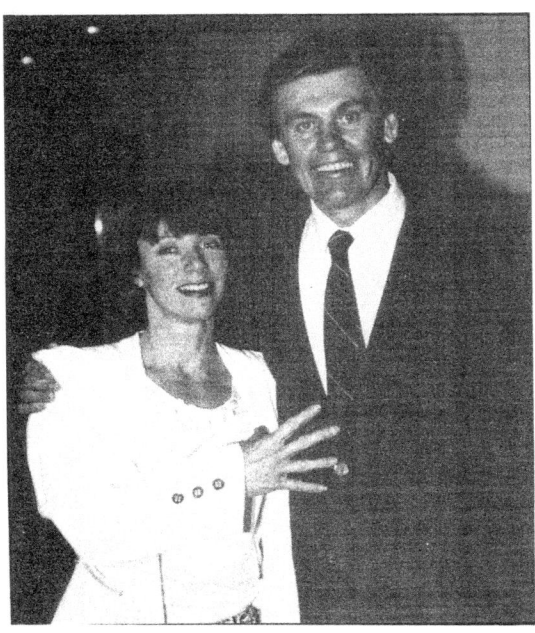

I'm pictured with Paula Crane who took some of the photos for this book.

Photo by Paula Crane

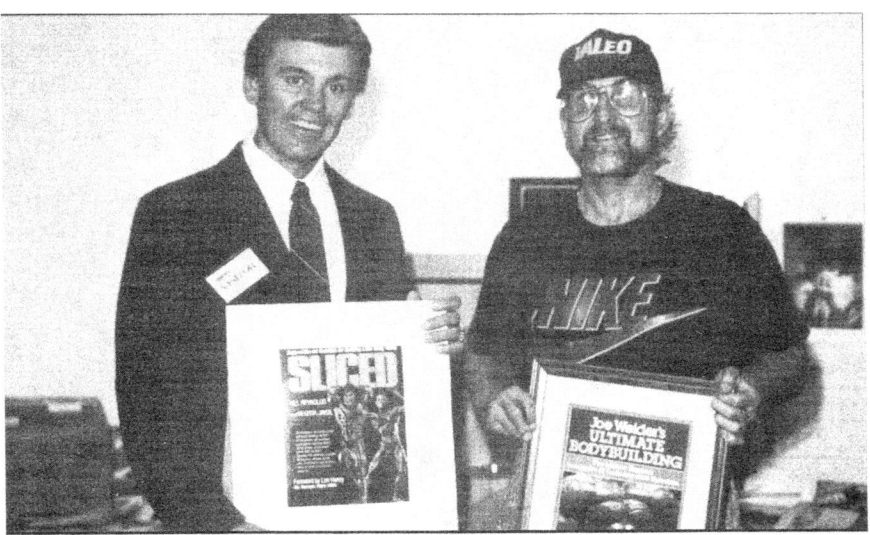

I am pictured with the onetime Editor of Flex Magazine, Bill Reynolds who is the author of numerous books. Bill has since passed on.

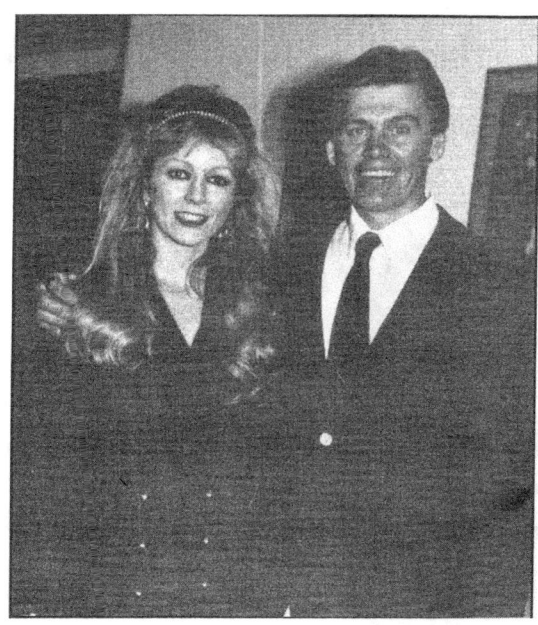

I am pictured with Joe Weider's former secretary Lisa Kenney.

Photo by Paula Crane

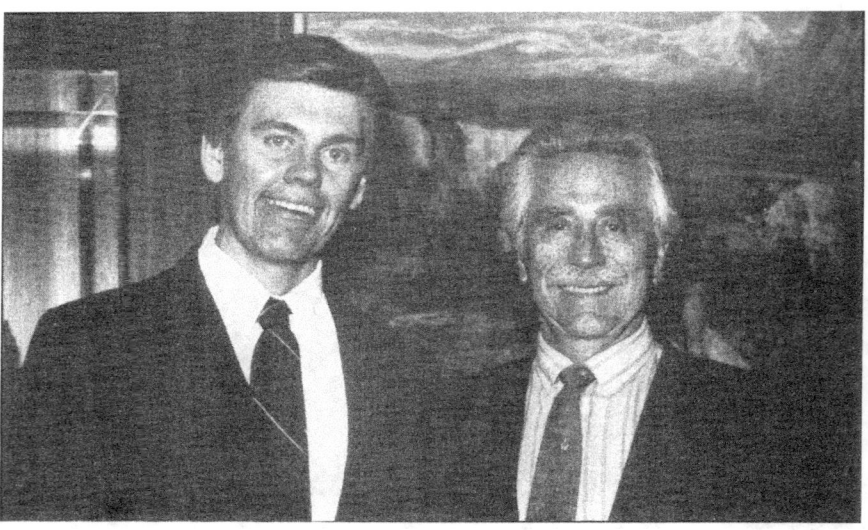

I'm pictured with Joe Weider, founder and former publisher of Muscle & Fitness Magazine. I thanked Joe for all the help he gave me with my mail order business and for the publicity he gave me in Muscle and Fitness. Joe will be greatly missed.

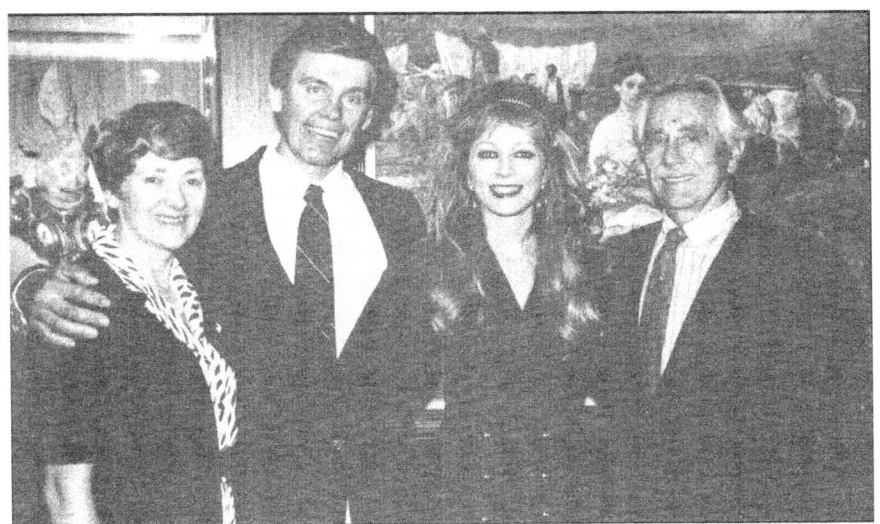

I am pictured with Joe Weider's former secretaries, Anneliese Leak and Lisa Kenney. Joe Weider was the founder and the publisher of Muscle and Fitness Magazine.

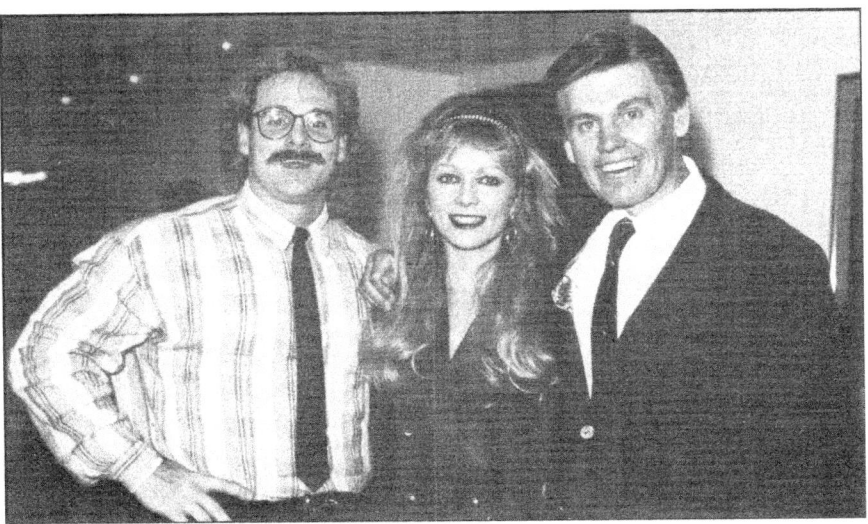

I'm pictured with former Editor of Muscle and Fitness Tom Deters D.C. and Lisa Kenney

Photo by Paula Crane

Train hard.

Eat the most nutritious foods.

Stay motivated.

Have patience and look for great results.

Best wishes,

Doug Bolus

Diet Tips

1. Avoid white sugar.

2. Avoid alcohol.

3. Eat a lot of fish.

4. Lot of fresh fruits and vegetables.

5. Relax after eating.

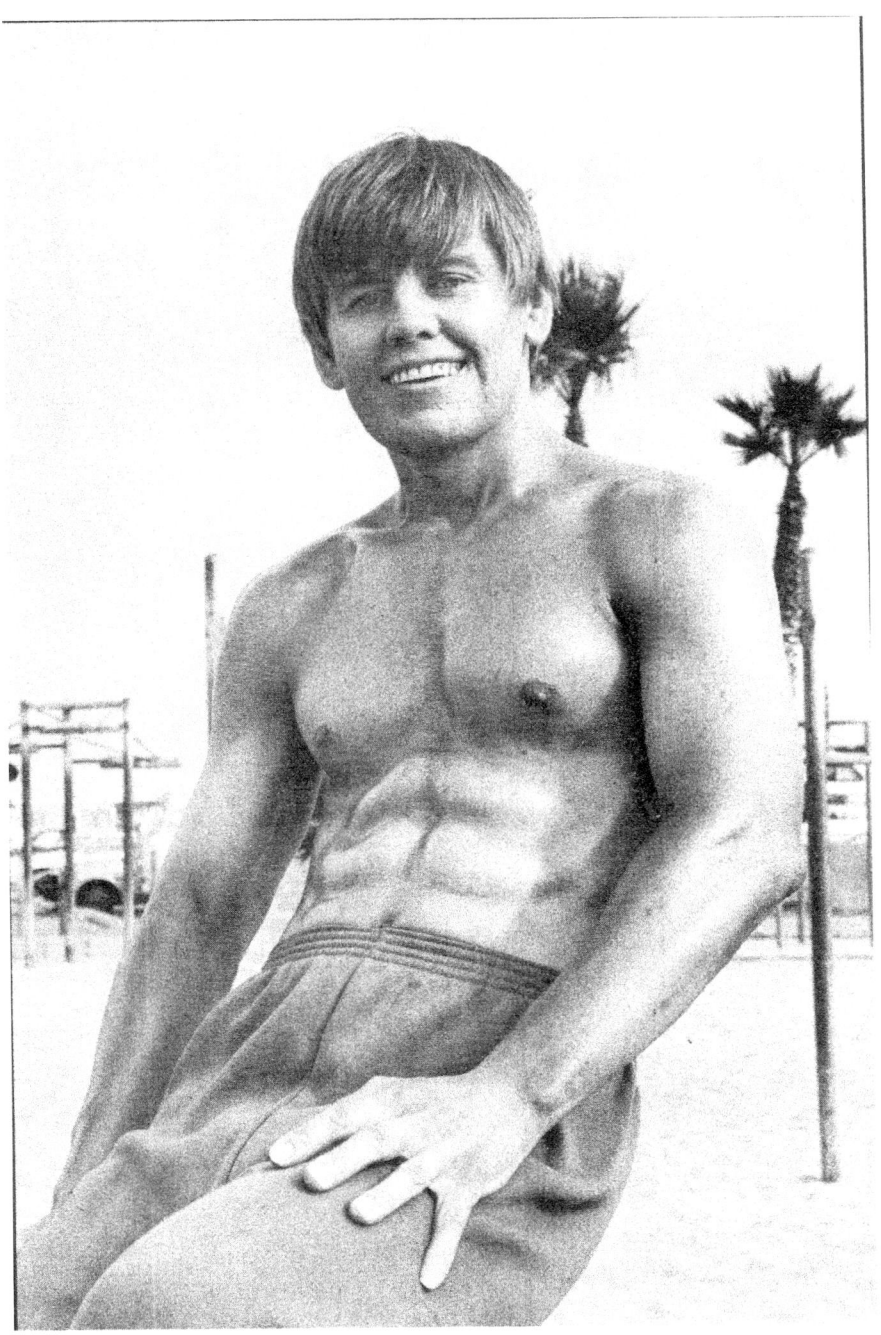

Relaxing at Muscle Beach in the early evening. Venice, California

Photo by Leon Bach

It's All Up To **YOU**.

NOW, start with the program!

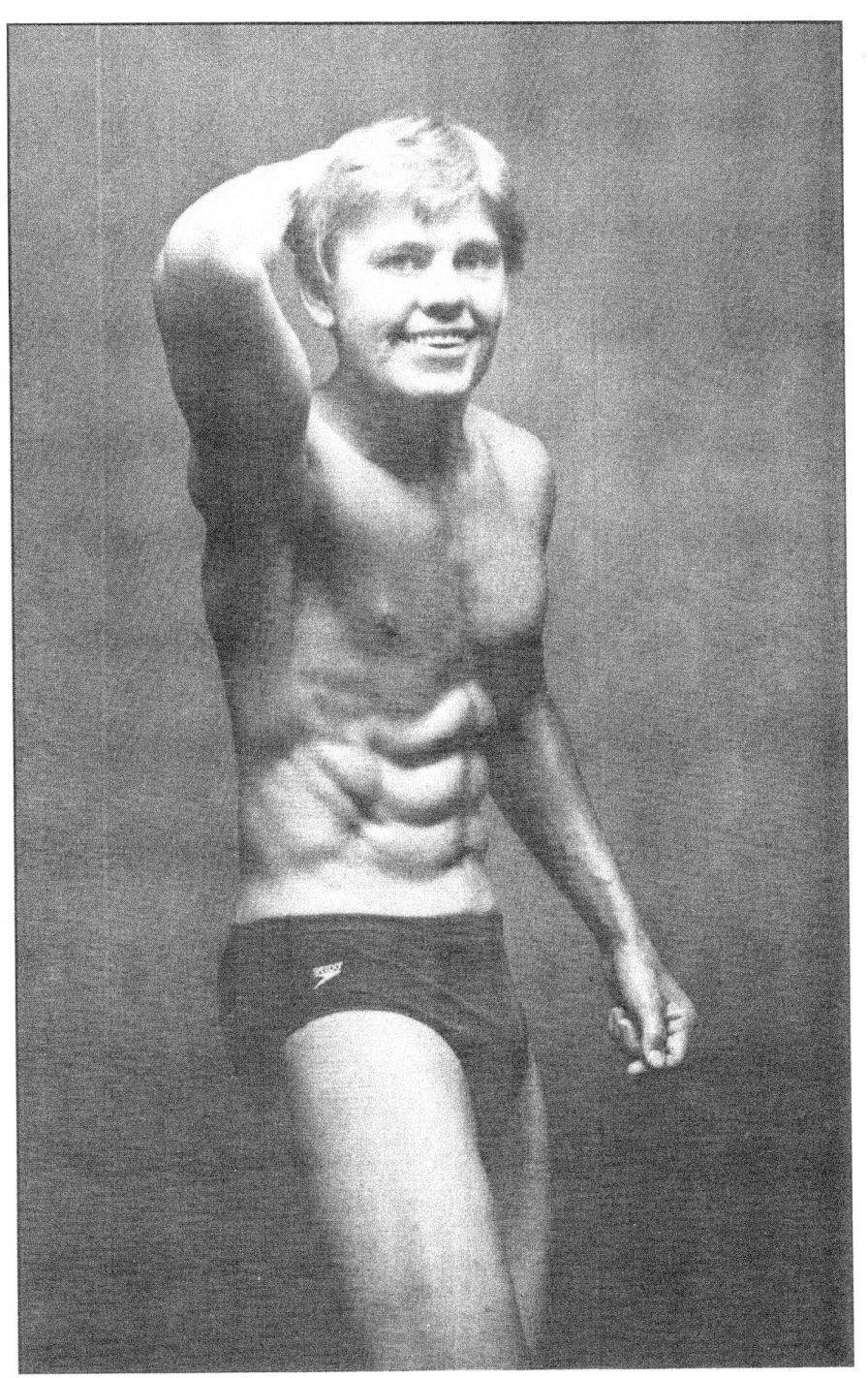